Intra-Uterine Insemination

Evidence-Based Guidelines for Daily Practice

T0383205

REPRODUCTIVE MEDICINE AND ASSISTED REPRODUCTIVE TECHNIQUES SERIES

David Gardner
University of Melbourne, Australia

Zeev Shoham
Kaplan Hospital, Rehovot, Israel

Kay Elder, Jacques Cohen
Human Preimplantation Embryo Selection, ISBN: 9780415399739

Michael Tucker, Juergen Liebermann
Vitrification in Assisted Reproduction, ISBN: 9780415408820

John D Aplin, Asgerally T Fazleabas, Stanley R Glasser, Linda C Giudice
The Endometrium, Second Edition, ISBN: 9780415385831

Nick Macklon, Ian Greer, Eric Steegers
Textbook of Periconceptional Medicine, ISBN: 9780415458924

Andrea Borini, Giovanni Coticchio
Preservation of Human Oocytes, ISBN: 9780415476799

Steven R Bayer, Michael M Alper, Alan S Penzias
The Boston IVF Handbook of Infertility, Third Edition, ISBN: 9781841848105

Ben Cohlen, Willem Ombelet
Intra-Uterine Insemination: Evidence-Based Guidelines for Daily Practice, ISBN: 9781841849881

Adam H. Balen
Infertility in Practice, Fourth Edition, ISBN: 9781841848495

Intra-Uterine Insemination

Evidence-Based Guidelines for Daily Practice

Edited by

Ben Cohlen, MD, PhD
Fertility Center Isala, Zwolle, The Netherlands

Willem Ombelet, MD, PhD
Institute for Fertility Technology, Ziekenhuis Oost Limburg, Genk, Belgium

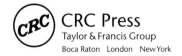

CRC Press
Taylor & Francis Group
Boca Raton   London   New York

CRC Press is an imprint of the
Taylor & Francis Group, an **informa** business

CRC Press
Taylor & Francis Group
6000 Broken Sound Parkway NW, Suite 300
Boca Raton, FL 33487-2742

© 2014 by Taylor & Francis Group, LLC
CRC Press is an imprint of Taylor & Francis Group, an Informa business

No claim to original U.S. Government works

Printed on acid-free paper
Version Date: 20130919

International Standard Book Number-13: 978-1-84184-988-1 (Paperback)

Library of Congress Cataloging-in-Publication Data

Intra-uterine insemination : evidence-based guidelines for daily practice / editors, Ben Cohlen, Willem Ombelet.
  p. ; cm. -- (Reproductive medicine and assisted reproductive techniques)
  Includes bibliographical references and index.
  ISBN 978-1-84184-988-1 (pbk. : alk. paper)
  I. Cohlen, Ben, 1963- editor of compilation. II. Ombelet, W. (Willem), editor of compilation. III. Series: Reproductive medicine & assisted reproductive techniques series.
  [DNLM: 1. Insemination, Artificial--methods. 2. Evidence-Based Medicine--standards. 3. Infertility--therapy. 4. Treatment Outcome. WQ 208]

  RG134
  618.1'78--dc23   2013036751

Visit the Taylor & Francis Web site at
http://www.taylorandfrancis.com

and the CRC Press Web site at
http://www.crcpress.com

Printed and bound by CPI Group (UK) Ltd, Croydon, CR0 4YY

Contents

Contributors

Ashok Agarwal
Center for Reproductive Medicine
Glickman Urological and Kidney Institute
Cleveland Clinic
Cleveland, Ohio

Alexandra J. Bensdorp
Center for Reproductive Medicine
Academic Medical Center
University of Amsterdam
Amsterdam, The Netherlands

Lars Björndahl
Center for Andrology and Sexual Medicine
Karolinska University Hospital
Karolinska Institutet, Huddinge
Stockholm, Sweden

Jacky Boivin
Cardiff University School of Psychology
Cardiff, United Kingdom

Carolien M. Boomsma
Department of Reproductive Medicine and
    Gynecology
University Medical Center–Utrecht
Utrecht, The Netherlands

Jan Bosteels
Department of Obstetrics and Gynecology
Imelda Hospital
Bonheiden, Belgium

Anne Brewaeys
Department of Developmental Psychology
Free University Brussels
Brussels, Belgium

Frank J.M. Broekmans
Department of Women and Baby
University Medical Center–Utrecht
Utrecht, The Netherlands

Michael de Brucker
Center for Reproductive Medicine
Free University
Brussels, Belgium

Rosario Buxaderas
Department of Obstetrics and Gynecology
Institut Universitari Quiron-Dexeus
Barcelona, Spain

Stuart Campbell
The Center for Reproduction and Advanced
    Technology
Create Health Clinic
London, United Kingdom

Astrid E.P. Cantineau
University Medical Center
Groningen, The Netherlands

Ben Cohlen
Fertility Center Isala
Zwolle, The Netherlands

Beatriz Corcostegui
Human Reproduction Unit
Hospital de Cruces
Baracaldo, Vizcaya, Spain

Lorena Crisol
Human Reproduction Unit
Hospital de Cruces
Baracaldo, Vizcaya, Spain

Inge M. Custers
Center for Reproductive Medicine
Academic Medical Center
University of Amsterdam
Amsterdam, The Netherlands

Nathalie Dhont
Genk Institute for Fertility Technology
Department of Obstetrics and Gynecology
Genk, Belgium

Thomas D'Hooghe
Leuven University Fertility Center
University Hospitals–Leuven
Leuven, Belgium

Irene Dimitriadis
MGH Fertility Center
Massachusetts General Hospital
Boston, Massachusetts

Ahmet Erdem
Department of Obstetrics and Gynecology
Gazi University School of Medicine
Ankara, Turkey

Antonia Exposito
Human Reproduction Unit
Hospital de Cruces
Baracaldo, Vizcaya, Spain

Nicolás Garrido
Instituto Universitario IVI Valencia
Universidad de Valencia
Valencia, Spain

Alaa Hamada
Center for Reproductive Medicine
Glickman Urological and Kidney Institute
Cleveland Clinic
Cleveland, Ohio

Carin Huyser
Department of Obstetrics and Gynecology
University of Pretoria
Steve Biko Academic Hospital
Arcadia, South Africa

Jarl A. Kahn
Fertility Clinic
Telemark County Hospital
Porsgrunn, Norway

Femke P.A.L. Kop
Center for Reproductive Medicine
Academic Medical Center
University of Amsterdam
Amsterdam, The Netherlands

Thinus Kruger
Reproductive Biology Unit
Department of Obstetrics and Gynecology
Stellenbosch University and Tygerberg Hospital
Tygerberg, South Africa

Pratap Kumar
Department of Obstetrics and Gynecology
Kasturba Medical College
Manipal, India

Roberto Matorras
Human Reproduction Unit
Hospital de Cruces
Basque Country University
and
IVI Bilbao
Baracaldo, Vizcaya, Spain

Roelof Menkveld
Department of Obstetrics and Gynecology
Tygerberg Academic Hospital and
    Stellenbosch University
Tygerberg, South Africa

Monique H. Mochtar
Center for Reproductive Medicine
Academic Medical Center
University of Amsterdam
Amsterdam, The Netherlands

Ben Willem Mol
Department of Obstetrics and Gynaecology
Academic Medical Center
University of Amsterdam
Amsterdam, The Netherlands

Lobke M. Moolenaar
Center for Reproductive Medicine
Academic Medical Center
University of Amsterdam
Amsterdam, The Netherlands

Geeta Nargund
St George's Hospital
London, United Kingdom
and
The Center for Reproduction and Advanced
    Technology
Create Health Clinic
London, United Kingdom

Diane de Neubourg
Leuven University Fertility Center
University Hospitals–Leuven
Leuven, Belgium

Martine Nijs
The Geertgen Foundation
Fertility Treatment Center
Elsendorp, The Netherlands

Sergio Oehninger
Department of Obstetrics and Gynecology
The Jones Institute for Reproductive Medicine
Eastern Virginia Medical School
Norfolk, Virginia

Willem Ombelet
Department of Obstetrics and Gynecology
Genk Institute for Fertility Technology
Genk, Belgium

Bonnie Patel
Department of Obstetrics and Gynecology
Greenville Hospital System University Medical
    Center
Greenville, South Carolina

Antonio Pellicer
Instituto Universitario IVI Valencia
Universidad de Valencia
Hospital Universitari i Politécnic la Fe
Valencia, Spain

Guido Pennings
Bioethics Institute Ghent (BIG)
Department of Philosophy and Moral Science
Ghent University
Ghent, Belgium

John C. Petrozza
Division of Reproductive Medicine and IVF
MGH Fertility Center
Massachusetts General Hospital
Harvard Medical School
Boston, Massachusetts

Olga Ramón
Human Reproduction Unit
Hospital de Cruces
Baracaldo, Vizcaya, Spain

William E. Roudebush
Department of Obstetrics and Gynecology
Greenville Hospital System–University Medical
    Center
Greenville, South Carolina
and
Department of Biomedical Sciences
University of South Carolina School of
    Medicine–Greenville
Greenville, South Carolina

Hasan N. Sallam
Obstetrics and Gynecology
University of Alexandria in Egypt
Alexandria, Egypt

Vasileios Sarafis
The Center for Reproduction and Advanced
    Technology
Create Health Clinic
London, United Kingdom

Jan Willem van der Steeg
Jeroen Bosch Ziekenhuis
Department of Obstetrics and Gynecology
's-Hertogenbosch, The Netherlands

Pieternel Steures
Sint Elisabeth Ziekenhuis
Department of Obstetrics and Gynecology
Tilburg, The Netherlands

Linda M. Street
Department of Obstetrics and Gynecology
Greenville Hospital System–University Medical
    Center
Greenville, South Carolina

Arne Sunde
Fertility Clinic
St. Olav's University Hospital
Trondheim, Norway

Petra de Sutter
Department of Reproductive Medicine
University Hospital–Ghent
Ghent, Belgium

Herman Tournaye
Center for Reproductive Medicine
Free University
Brussels, Belgium

Rosa Tur
Department of Obstetrics and Gynecology
Institut Universitari Quiron-Dexeus
Barcelona, Spain

Sheryl Vanderpoel
Department of Reproductive Health and
    Research
World Health Organization
Geneva, Switzerland

Fulco van der Veen
Center for Reproductive Medicine
Academic Medical Center
University of Amsterdam
Amsterdam, The Netherlands

Egbert te Velde
Department of Public Health
Erasmus University MC
Rotterdam, The Netherlands
and
Reproductive Medicine
Utrecht University
Utrecht, The Netherlands

Chris Verhaak
Radboud University
Nijmegen Medical Center
Nijmegen, The Netherlands

Benny Verheyden
Center for Reproductive Medicine
University Hospital Antwerp
Antwerp, Belgium

Harold Verhoeve
Department of Obstetrics and Gynecology
Academic Medical Center
University of Amsterdam
Amsterdam, The Netherlands

Bradley J. Van Voorhis
Department of Obstetrics and Gynecology
University of Iowa Carver College of Medicine
Iowa City, Iowa

Janne-Meije van Weert
Department of Obstetrics and Gynecology
Academic Medical Center
University of Amsterdam
Amsterdam, The Netherlands

Felicia Yarde
Department of Women and Baby
University Medical Center–Utrecht
Utrecht, The Netherlands

Evidence Evaluation

The levels of evidence used in the *Statements* in this text are as follows:

1a	Systematic review and meta-analysis of randomized controlled trials
1b	At least one randomized controlled trial
2a	At least one well-designed controlled study without randomization
2b	At least one other type of well-designed quasi-experimental study
3	Well-designed non-experimental descriptive studies, such as comparative studies, correlation studies, or case studies
4	Expert committee reports or opinions and/or clinical experience of respected authorities

The strength of evidence is graded as follows for the *Recommendations* (guidelines) in this text:

A	Directly based on Level 1 evidence
B	Directly based on Level 2 evidence or extrapolated recommendation from Level 1 evidence
C	Directly based on Level 3 evidence or extrapolated recommendation from either Level 1 or 2 evidence
D	Directly based on Level 4 evidence or extrapolated recommendation from either Level 1, 2, or 3 evidence
GPP	Good practice point (GPP)

1

General Introduction to Intra-Uterine Insemination (IUI) as a Treatment for Subfertility: The Impressions of an Old-Timer

Egbert te Velde

During the end of the 1980s, we decided that *the clinical value of intra-uterine insemination (IUI)* would be one of the research themes of our department for the next 10 years. A few years later I was lucky to have an ambitious, young fertility doctor on my team who was willing to take up this subject; his name was Ben Cohlen. These were the exciting years of the introduction of Evidence-based Medicine (EBM) in reproductive medicine altering infertility treatment "from cookery to science."[1] We were keen to apply the principles of EBM in our research. Obviously, the ultimate aim of IUI is the occurrence of a live birth pregnancy but since the publication of John Collins' milestone paper "Treatment-Independent Pregnancy among Infertile Couples" in the *New England Journal of Medicine*[2] we were very much aware of the fact that a spontaneously occurring live birth pregnancy is not at all a rare event among so-called infertile couples, and certainly not among those who have an indication for IUI when the female and male partner must have patent tubes and fair sperm qualities. How to find out whether the available interventions—the IUI, the so-called ovarian hyperstimulation (OH), or the combination of both (IUI/OH)—would be more effective than the natural chance to conceive? In order to unravel the puzzle of these four *unknowns* and assess the effect of each, we had to resolve four different equations by randomized controlled trials (RCT), and so we depicted our magic square of comparisons of which this figure (Figure 1.1) was the very first version drawn by hand before the era of Windows and PowerPoint.

In Belgium there was another rising star in the firmament of reproductive medicine who organized the so-called "Andrology-in-the-Nineties" conferences in the city of Genk. These conferences soon became well known and influential because of their excellent organization, the international scope, and the informal atmosphere. The name of this star was Willem Ombelet. He invited me to give a lecture on "Intra-Uterine Insemination: An Update" at the 1993 conference, which I did on behalf of Ben Cohlen and Roel van Kooij, our embryologist-andrologist. I presented there the square of comparisons of the figure and the available RCTs, which fitted in these comparisons. During the following years it was always Ben Cohlen who would give the lectures on this subject. In addition, he was the first author of various publications, which would result in his thesis in 1997 "Intra-Uterine Insemination for Treating Male Subfertility and Cervical Hostility," in which some methodological problems were also tackled. We demonstrated for example, that a crossover design has many practical advantages over a parallel design in cycle-related fertility research while being as accurate as a parallel design.[3] Unfortunately, the crossover design was banned by the EBM community and we were forced to use a parallel design for our research in order to get it published.

In 1998, I was invited by the *NEJM* to write a commentary on an article entitled "Efficacy of Superovulation and Intra-Uterine Insemination in the Treatment of Infertility,"[4] which I did on behalf of Ben Cohlen.[5] Although, being a monument of EBM including almost 1000 couples of 10 clinical sites evenly randomized over the four comparisons shown in the figure, we criticized the contents of the paper on two aspects. First, timed intracervical insemination with prepared semen was adopted by the authors as the baseline control tacitly assuming that it had the same success chance as natural intercourse. The detailed information given in the material and methods section of the Guzick article[4]

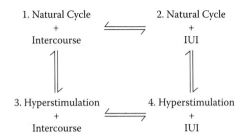

FIGURE 1.1   Comparisons to be made to (dis)prove the beneficial effects of IUI, OH, or the combination of both.

allowed us to demonstrate that the natural pregnancy chance of the rest cycles in between the treatment cycles was noticeably higher than the intracervical insemination cycles: my interest in the paramount importance of the baseline control was aroused. In addition, we were concerned about the high multiple pregnancy rate in the study arm where the results of ovarian stimulation and IUI were assessed. We argued that IUI should never become a first line treatment of infertility unless this rate would be much lower.

Ben Cohlen and Willem Ombelet—two young and promising fertility doctors some 20 years ago—have become authorities in the field of reproductive medicine. They are the editors of *Intra-Uterine Insemination: Evidence-Based Guidelines for Daily Practice.* The two editors aim to make this book a "comprehensive evidence-based book with guidelines for daily practice." Did they succeed? I will try to answer this question in the following paragraphs.

The Appropriate Baseline Control

The insight that clinical medicine until the 1970s was largely based on authorities' opinions, intuition, and subjective judgment was a big step forward and indeed the EBM crusade is a heroic attempt to move from "cookery to science."[1] However, the progress of science is a complex process of contradicting opinions and continuous debate, the truth is covered by rocks and jungle and, accordingly, progress in EBM usually goes by little steps and is certainly much slower than I had envisaged 20 years ago. Moreover, observations from other studies may change our opinions and may cast doubt on what has been reached after years of laborious and arduous EBM research.

An example of such an experience is related to the question of what the most appropriate baseline control in IUI research should be. The most common one applied so far is timed intercourse (TI), using urinary or serum LH testing for advising the couple when to have intercourse, that is one day after the LH rise on the perceived day of ovulation. Twenty years ago, I belonged to the fertility specialists who took it for granted that this was the most appropriate control. However, information on the fertile window of the menstrual cycle, and timing and frequency of intercourse that has emerged since that time[6–9] indicates that the fertile window of the menstrual cycle precedes the day of ovulation by 5 to 6 days and that the likelihood of pregnancy is highest when intercourse occurs 2 days before ovulation. Intercourse at the day of ovulation is less effective and success rates are almost zero on the day after ovulation. A coital frequency of three times during the week of the fertile window is optimal but a frequency of twice during that week is almost as effective. However, a reduction in the frequency from twice to once a week results in a 40% reduction of the success chance. According to these findings, TI in IUI research is advised on a day of the cycle when the chance of conceiving is considerably reduced. Moreover, intercourse is usually not advised on other days than after the LH surge, thus it probably often takes place once during the fertile window or not at all. The question arises if the reported success of IUI, whether or not combined with OH, is (partly) to be explained by the artificially low chance of pregnancy after TI as compared to the natural situation when couples want to have a child and are keen to become pregnant. It is noteworthy in this respect that in the only two research papers where expectant management (EM) was adopted as the control of IUI, no effect was seen of clomiphene citrate stimulation and IUI in natural cycles[10] and of

IUI in combination with mild gonadotrophin stimulation in couples with an intermediate prognosis.[11] In couples with an isolated cervical factor, IUI in natural cycles seemed to improve the pregnancy chances of EM, although statistical significance was not reached.[12] The question is justified whether or not many of the results, conclusions, and advice of IUI research in the past as collected in some *Cochrane Reviews*, would have been different if EM instead of TI was adopted as the baseline control. This also raises the question of whether the performance of IUI for moderate or even severe male subfertility in natural cycles would be more effective if inseminations were to be performed twice during the optimal days of the fertile window instead of only once at the perceived day of ovulation. In women with a more or less regular cycle pattern, this is a feasible possibility.

In Chapter 4 this view is clearly expressed where it is stated "To (dis)prove a beneficial effect of IUI this technique should be compared with expected management in a well-described population in a large randomized trial." In Chapter 3, this vision is not explicitly stated, but implicitly the authors seem to embrace this stand when they write "IUI should only be offered to a couple if the success rate after IUI clearly exceeds the probability of a treatment independent pregnancy in that couple." This undoubtedly is related to the emphasis in that chapter on the importance of prediction rules by which the individual, treatment-independent prognosis of a live birth pregnancy can be calculated. "It is of major importance," they state, "to explain to the couple at their first visit the prognostic approach. Their prognostic profile is being calculated and based on this prognosis the best treatment policy will be determined." In my opinion, EM as the control for measuring the effect of possible treatment options and the assessment of the couple's prognosis in order to decide whether or not to treat should be the keystones of future IUI research. These insights, in my opinion, are some of the great merits of this book.

Progress in Evidence-Based IUI Research

Progress in evidence-based IUI research may imply less instead of more certainty about its possible beneficial effects. This is illustrated by the conclusions of a *Cochrane Review* about IUI in male subfertility in 2000[13] and one in 2007.[14] In both reviews, the first author of Chapter 4 was involved. In 2000, the conclusion was:

> Intra-uterine insemination offers couples with male subfertility benefit over timed intercourse, both in natural cycles and in cycles with OH. In the case of a severe semen defect IUI in natural cycles should be the treatment of first choice. The value of OH needs to be further investigated in RCTs. Mild ovarian hyperstimulation with gonadotrophins is advised in cases with less severe semen defects (for instance: average total motile sperm concentration >10 million).

In 2007, the conclusion was:

> There was insufficient evidence of effectiveness to recommend or advise against IUI with or without OH above TI, or vice versa. Large, high quality randomized controlled trials, comparing IUI with or without OH with pregnancy rate per couple as the main outcome of interest are lacking. There is a need for such trials since firm conclusions cannot be drawn yet.

Undoubtedly, more RCTs were available in the last review but their results were different. Seemingly firm conclusions from the past had to be withdrawn. This example illustrates the kind of progress EBM has to go through, requiring sometimes taking a step backward.

Questions Resolved?

Many questions for which there was no clear answer some 20 years ago seem to have been resolved at first sight. However, sometimes the answer is less straightforward when looking more carefully. I give an example related to this important question: should we inseminate once or twice per stimulated cycle?

The 2009 *Cochrane Review* performed in 2009 by the authors of Chapter 14 in which couples with unexplained and mild male subfertility (total sperm count >10 million) were included, gives a direct answer: two inseminations result in higher pregnancy rates compared with single IUI. But then the considerations and deliberations, so typical for EBM reviews, start. In this example, the conclusions reached were mainly based on the results of one large study in which only couples with mild male subfertility were included. In the studies with unexplained subfertility, only a single act of IUI resulted in the same success rate as double IUI. In spite of the fact that the authors argue somewhere else that the mild male subfertility group is to be considered as unexplained subfertility, the concluding statements of Chapter 14 are now: "Double IUI does not result in higher pregnancy rates compared with single IUI treatment in women with unexplained subfertility undergoing ovarian hyperstimulation" (Level of Evidence 1a) and "Double IUI results in higher pregnancy rates compared with single IUI in couples with male factor subfertility" (Level of Evidence 1a). It is not unlikely that in the next survey on this subject conclusions will change again. As stated above: this is progress in EBM.

Unexpected Results

Sometimes amazingly unexpected results and conclusions have been reached. Who would have thought "10 to 15 minutes immobilization subsequent to IUI, with or without ovarian stimulation, significantly improves cumulative ongoing pregnancy rates and live birth rates" (Chapter 16)? Does that partly explain the success of normal intercourse when partners usually remain *immobilized* for a while after the act of love? And what about the finding that female obesity is a favorable prognostic factor in IUI treatment (Chapter 8)?

Useful Observations and Recommendations

Several chapters of the book contain useful observations and recommendations for daily practice, which were unknown or less evident 20 years ago. I mention a few:

- Premature LH surges quite often occur in gonadotrophin-stimulated cycles and may adversely impact the results of IUI. However, the addition of GnRH antagonists in IUI cycles with mild ovarian hyperstimulation has been shown not to increase live birth rates (Chapter 17).
- When the decision for IUI has been taken do not stop after three cycles. It is worthwhile to continue for six, possibly nine cycles (Chapter 12).
- With regard to sperm preparation techniques (Chapter 10)—gradient, swim-up, or wash techniques—the discussion is closed for the time being with the statement "concerning pregnancy rates after IUI: there is no clear evidence which technique is superior," with the additional remark by the authors that high quality RCTs comparing the effectiveness of these techniques are still warranted. But that is a remark often added on: almost never is it possible to include enough good studies in meta-analyses and reviews to give really strong statements.

Promising Developments, Which May Improve the Results of IUI in the Future

- Several small randomized trials found a significant benefit of the use of luteal support with vaginally applied progesterone in stimulated IUI cycles (Chapter 18). However, before this drug is to be introduced in IUI programs, the results of large RCTs have to confirm these first promising results.
- Several novel sperm selection methods have recently been developed for IVF and Intra Cytoplasmic Sperm Injection (ICSI). These methods aim at isolating mature, structurally intact and nonapoptotic spermatozoa with high DNA integrity (Chapter 21). Their value for IUI sperm preparation still needs to be demonstrated.

- Human sperm prepared for IUI using a sperm wash medium supplemented with platelet-activating factor (PAF) resulted in considerably increased pregnancy rates (Chapter 20). These results are based on two studies performed in 2004 and 2005, and as far as I know, have not been repeated by others.

What Is the Future of IUI?

The authors of Chapter 22 are most explicit in their statements on future developments:

> As we look to the future, it is clear that there may be shifting paradigms as to the most cost-effective treatment strategy for infertile couples. In recent years, there has been a steady increase in pregnancy rates with IVF. Similar increases have not been achieved with IUI treatments. Indeed several recent studies modeling outcomes and costs have concluded that moving directly to IVF may be more cost-effective than starting with IUI cycles for unexplained and mild male factor infertility. If the singleton delivery rate per cycle can be improved with single embryo transfer, IVF may become the favored first line treatment for most causes of infertility.

and "…, the use of OH using gonadotrophin injections and IUI as an intermediate step prior to IVF has to be questioned." If strict elective single embryo transfer (eSET) and the transfer of additional frozen-thawed embryos in subsequent natural cycles will become the standard in IVF/ICSI strategy as often is suggested and already successfully practiced in some places, IVF may well become the first line treatment for all infertile couples. A satisfactory singleton live birth rate with almost no multiples is assured with such a strategy. Data presented in Chapter 17 indicate that twin pregnancy rates of 10% are common after IUI/OH in the Netherlands and the last ESHRE Monitoring Consortium reported an almost 12% twin delivery rate and 0.5% triplets in 2007 in Europe.[15] IUI in combination with OH may only be able to compete with eSET if multiple pregnancy rates can be considerably reduced. Is that conceivable?

Data given in Chapters 26 and 27 indicate that both the pregnancy chance and the multiple pregnancy risk are more dependent on the number of stimulated follicles than on the kind or dose of OH used, although both obviously are strongly related. A review article often referred to in these and other chapters entitled "The Influence of the Number of Follicles on Pregnancy Rates in Intra-Uterine Insemination with Ovarian Stimulation: A Meta-Analysis" by Van Rumste et al.[16] compares total and multiple pregnancy rates after mono-follicular and bi-follicular stimulation. The pregnancy rates were 7.4 and 13.4% per cycle after mono-follicular and bi-follicular growth, respectively. However, the multiple pregnancy rates in case of pregnancy are 3.7% after mono-follicular growth and 17% after bi-follicular growth. If these numbers are representative—there were only five studies for the comparison just mentioned—the last figure seems unacceptably high. Consequently, one should only perform IUI in case of mono-follicular growth and not strive for two growing follicles, which is in line with modern IVF practice where the routine transfer of two embryos is also not acceptable anymore. Is this the future of IUI? Or will there only be a place for a short initial period of some clomiphene citrate-stimulated IUI cycles directly followed by IVF, which is the scheme mentioned in Chapter 22 as one of the most cost-effective options?

Conclusion

Did the editors succeed in making this book a "comprehensive evidence-based book with guidelines for daily practice" as is their aim?

Apart from practical advice and guidelines for the daily practice of IUI, I think they did more. This book also inspires a reader like me to contemplate the nuances, problems, and (lack of) progress of infertility treatment in particular and reproductive medicine in general.

REFERENCES

1. Vandekerckhove P., O'Donovan P.A., Lilford R.J., and Harada T.W. 1993. Infertility treatment: From cookery to science. The epidemiology of randomized controlled trials. *Br J Obstet Gynaecol* 100:1005–1036. Review.

2. Collins J.A., Wrixon W., Janes L.B., and Wilson E.H. 1983. Treatment-independent pregnancy among infertile couples. *N Engl J Med* 309:1201–1206.

3. Cohlen B.J., te Velde E.R., Looman C.W., Eijckemans R., and Habbema J.D.F. 1998. Crossover or parallel design in infertility trials? The discussion continues. *Fertil Steril* 69:40–45.

4. Guzick D.S., Carson S.A., Coutifaris C., Overstreet J.W., Factor-Litvak P., Hill J.A., Mastroianni L., Buster J.E., Nakajima S.T., Vogel D.L., and Canfield R.E. 1999. Efficacy of superovulation and intrauterine insemination in the treatment of infertility. *N Engl J Med* 340:177–183.

5. te Velde E.R. and Cohlen B.J. 1999. The management of infertility. *N Engl J Med* 224–226.

6. Wilcox A.J., Weinberg C.R., and Baird D. 1995. Timing of sexual intercourse in relation to ovulation. *N Engl J Med* 333:1517–1521.

7. Wilcox A.J., Dunson D.B., Weinberg C.R., Trussell J., and Day Baird D. 2001. Likelihood of conception with a single act of intercourse: Providing benchmark rates for assessment of post-coital contraceptives. *Contraception* 63:211–215.

8. Stanford J.B. and Dunson D.B. 2007. Effects of sexual intercourse patterns in time to pregnancy studies. *Am J Epidemiol* 165:1088–1095.

9. ASRM. 2008. Optimizing natural fertility. *Fertil Steril* 90: S1–6.

10. Bhattacharya S., Harrild K., Mollison J., Wordsworth S., Tay C., and Harrold A. 2008. Clomifene citrate or unstimulated intrauterine insemination compared with expectant management for unexplained infertility: Pragmatic randomised controlled trial. *BMJ* 7(337):a716.

11. Steures P., Van der Steeg J.W., Hompes P.G., Habbema J.D., Eijkemans M.J., Broekmans F.J., Verhoeve H.R., Bossuyt P.M., Van der Veen F., and Mol B.W. 2006. Intrauterine insemination with controlled ovarian hyperstimulation versus expectant management for couples with unexplained subfertility and an intermediate prognosis: A randomised clinical trial. *Lancet* 3.

12. Steures P., Van der Steeg J.W., Hompes P.G., Bossuyt P.M., Habbema J.D., Eijkemans M.J., Schols W.A., Burggraaff J.M., Van der Veen F., and Mol B.W. 2007. Effectiveness of intrauterine insemination in subfertile couples with an isolated cervical factor: A randomized clinical trial. *Fertil Steril* 88:1692–1696.

13. Cohlen B.J., Vandekerckhove P., te Velde E.R., and Habbema J.D. 2000. Timed intercourse versus intra-uterine insemination with or without ovarian hyperstimulation for subfertility in men. *Cochrane Database Syst Rev* (2):CD000360.

14. Bensdorp A.J., Cohlen B.J, Heineman M.J., and Vandekerckhove P. 2007. Intra-uterine insemination for male subfertility. *Cochrane Database Syst Rev* October 17;(4):CD000360.

15. de Mouzon J., Goossens V., Bhattacharya S., Castilla J.A., Ferraretti A.P., Korsak V., Kupka M., Nygren K.G., Andersen A.N., and European IVF-Monitoring (EIM), Consortium for the European Society on Human Reproduction and Embryology (ESHRE). 2012. Assisted reproductive technology in Europe. *Hum Reprod* 24:954–966.

16. Van Rumste M.M., Custers I.M., Van der Veen F., Van Wely M., Evers J.L., and Mol B.W. 2008. The influence of the number of follicles on pregnancy rates in intrauterine insemination with ovarian stimulation: A meta-analysis. *Hum Reprod Update* 6:563–570.

2

Diagnostic Work-Up before IUI

Janne-Meije van Weert, Harold Verhoeve, and Ben Willem Mol

The diagnostic work-up of a couple before intra-uterine insemination (IUI) should be limited to those tests that contribute to the prediction of effectiveness of IUI. In general, the indications for IUI are moderate semen deficiencies or longstanding unexplained subfertility, but these indications are more elaborately discussed in Chapter 4. Female age and duration of subfertility are the most important factors predicting IUI outcome, and for these, no tests are required.[1] Although semen quality and other female factors seem of lesser consequence, they do have some importance and will be discussed in this chapter.

A semen analysis is considered normal if the WHO criteria from 2010 are met, that is, when the volume is >1.5 ml, concentration is $> 15 \times 10^6$/ml, the total sperm count is $> 39 \times 10^6$, percentage motility is >40%, and normal morphology is >4%.[2] These WHO criteria have limited value in the prediction of a spontaneous pregnancy, but no value in the prediction of a pregnancy after IUI.[3] It is also important to realize that semen quality can differ considerably within one man over time,[4] so a second semen analysis should be performed if the first is abnormal. For the diagnosis of male subfertility, the total motile sperm count (TMSC) can be calculated from the semen analysis by multiplying volume (ml) × concentration ($.10^6$/ml) × progressive motility (%), and is helpful in identifying three crude groups of male subfertility. Mild male subfertility with a TMSC $> 3 \times 10^6$, moderate male subfertility with a TMSC $1–3 \times 10^6$, and severe male subfertility with a TMSC $< 1 \times 10^6$. These cut-off values are by no means strict, as there are no data from the literature that have sufficiently proved themselves, but they are an estimation based on the WHO criteria and the crude cut-off values for IUI, IVF, and ICSI. They are used in the Dutch gynecological and general practitioner guidelines. If male subfertility is diagnosed, semen preparation should be part of the fertility work-up to establish the so-called, postwash TMSC. In the mild and moderate group, IUI can be considered if the postwash TMSC lies between 0.8×10^6 and 5×10^6 motile spermatozoa (Table 2.2: LOE 2a).[3] This implicates that in the moderate male subfertility group IUI can seldom be performed, because there is an approximate loss of motile spermatozoa of 70% with preparation. The amount of motile spermatozoa after preparation depends on the preparation technique used. This will be discussed in Chapter 10. All in all, in the decision making whether IUI is a feasible option, female age and duration of subfertility should be taken into account.

To detect the presence of antisperm antibodies (ASA) in the semen, an immunobead test or antisperm antibodies (ASA) can be used. Whether these tests should be routinely performed has been debated, since the presence of ASA in semen does not predict the chance of a spontaneous pregnancy (LOE 2a).[5] Screening for ASA could, however, be of use before the start of IUI. If ASA are present, semen preparation with an additional medium can elute the antibodies from the acrosome region and lead to a better fertilization capacity of spermatozoa.[6]

Although the above stated tests can help to identify and classify male subfertility, there are as yet no validated instruments to help in the decision of which treatment is the most effective.

A postcoital test used to be part of the diagnostic work-up for subfertility. In this test, couples were asked to have intercourse in the fertile period, and 8 to 16 hours after coitus, mucus from the cervix was sampled and examined for the presence of motile spermatozoa. If spermatozoa were absent or nonmotile, the postcoital test was considered to be abnormal, and IUI in a natural cycle was recommended.

However, a recent randomized trial in isolated cervical factor subfertility (i.e., an abnormal PCT and no other cause for subfertility) showed no significant benefit of IUI compared with no treatment at 6 months follow-up (LOE 1b).[7] This study confirmed that the general policy to abandon the postcoital test in the fertility work-up is correct.

All women undergo a gynecological examination and usually an ultrasound as part of their general diagnostic work-up for subfertility. Causes for ovulatory problems should be investigated and corrected if possible. There is no evidence that in the presence of a regular cycle, ultrasound monitoring of the cycle adds to the diagnostic effectiveness of the work-up. In some women ultrasound may reveal visible hydro-salpinges or ovarian pathology. In order for IUI to be successful, the fallopian tubes should be patent. Tubal pathology is a common cause for in- or subfertility. The prevalence depends on the population studied and varies between primary, secondary, and tertiary study populations. Patient characteristics and the chlamydia antibody test (CAT) can help to differentiate between women who have a low or a high risk of bilateral tubal pathology (Table 2.1: LOE 2b).[8]

Diagnostic tests for tubal patency are usually planned as last tests in the work-up for subfertility. There are several reasons for postponement of these tests. First, they are invasive procedures that are uncomfortable to women. Second, they need to be planned and can generate healthcare costs. Third, complications such as infection or injury to the genital or internal organs can occur. And fourth, a planned invasive test may become unnecessary, because natural conception has occurred after the first consultation of a couple but before the planned diagnostic test has been performed.

Traditionally, hysterosalpingography (HSG) and diagnostic laparoscopy (DL) are performed, HSG being the first line test and DL the so-called gold standard or reference test. An alternative for DL is transvaginal hydrolaparoscopy (THL), which has a comparable diagnostic accuracy as DL, but can be performed in an outpatient setting without general anesthesia. Whether THL should replace HSG as a first line test is unknown.[9] In women at high risk, early tests may be warranted to exclude bilateral tubal pathology, whereas in women at low risk many tests would be required to detect one abnormality. Identification of those women at highest risk for bilateral tubal pathology is best obtained by combining the patient characteristics with CAT and HSG results (Table 2.1: LOE 2a).[10]

The cost-effectiveness of different diagnostic strategies for tubal pathology was recently examined in a Markov analytic model. Six different scenarios for tubal testing were compared and outcome measures were cumulative live-birth rates and costs per couple at 3 years from the start of unprotected intercourse. The model showed that the most cost-effective scenario is to perform no diagnostic tubal tests until the age of 30 years, and from the age of 40 the prevalence of bilateral tubal pathology was of no influence on the outcome. The threshold value for the prevalence of bilateral tubal disease at which direct treatment (i.e., IVF) became more cost-effective than delaying treatment by one year declined gradually from 95% at the age of 31 to 10% at the age of 39, indicating that even in the younger woman at very high risk of tubal pathology, it is not cost-effective to plan a diagnostic tubal patency test early in the fertility work-up. Presence and treatment of minimal or mild endometriosis did not influence the outcome. If tubal tests were performed, HSG and DL for those women with bilateral tubal pathology at HSG, followed by treatment according to findings, was more cost-effective than DL (Table 2.2: LOE 2b).[11]

TABLE 2.1

Statements of Chapter 2

Statement	Level of Evidence (LOE)
If antisperm antibodies are present, semen preparation for IUI with an additional medium to elude the antibodies leads to a better fertilization capacity of spermatozoa	2a
The postcoital test should not be part of the fertility work-up	1b
The medical history can differentiate between women at low or at high risk for bilateral tubal pathology	2b
Identification of those women at highest risk for bilateral tubal pathology is best obtained by combining the patient characteristics with CAT and HSG results	2a
Routinely testing for tubal pathology is not cost-effective	2b

TABLE 2.2

Recommendations of Chapter 2

Recommendation	Grade Strength
IUI should be considered if the postwash TMSC lies between 0.8–5.0 million motile sperm	A
Screening for antisperm antibodies before the start of IUI could be of use	B
If tubal tests are performed, HSG followed by a diagnostic laparoscopy in case HSG shows no tubal patency is more cost-effective than diagnostic laparoscopy	B

When the advice is not to perform tubal tests, it is obvious that this should be discussed with the woman.

In summary, although a thorough history of female factors including duration of subfertility, the menstrual cycle, and risk assessment for presence of tubal pathology should be leading the decision making, a semen analysis should not be left out. Even for this test, interpretation is difficult, as exact criteria to distinguish the indication for IUI, IVF, or ICSI in male subfertility are lacking. A mixed agglutination reaction (MAR) might add to that diagnosis. Tubal tests are often routinely done, but in the absence of risk factors for tubal pathology they are of limited value (see Table 2.2).

REFERENCES

1. Steures P., Van der Steeg J.W., Mol B.W., Eijkemans M.J., Van der Veen F., Habbema J.D., Hompes P.G., Bossuyt P.M., Verhoeve H.R., Van Kasteren Y.M., Van Dop P.A., CECERM (Collaborative Effort in Clinical Evaluation in Reproductive Medicine). 2004. Prediction of an ongoing pregnancy after intrauterine insemination. *Fertil Steril.* 82:45–51.
2. World Health Organization. 2010. *Laboratory Manual for the Examination of Human Semen and Semen-Cervical Mucus Interaction*, 5th ed. New York: Cambridge University Press. 287.
3. Van Weert J.M., Repping S., Van Voorhis B., Bossuyt P., Van der Veen F., Mol B.W. 2004. The performance of the post-wash total motile sperm count at the time of intrauterine insemination from the prediction of pregnancy: A meta-analysis. *Fertil Steril.* 82:612–20.
4. Leushuis E., Van der Steeg J.W., Steures P., Repping S., Bossuyt P.M., Blankenstein M.A., Mol B.W., Van der Veen F., Hompes P.G. 2010. Reproducibility and reliability of repeated semen analyses in male partners of subfertile couples. *Fertil Steril.* 94:2631–5.
5. Leushuis E., Van der Steeg J.W., Steures P., Repping S., Schöls W., Van der Veen F., Mol B.W., Hompes P.G. 2009. Immunoglobulin G antisperm antibodies and prediction of spontaneous pregnancy. *Fertil Steril.* 92:1659–65.
6. Van Weert J.M., Repping S., Van der Steeg J.W., Steures P., Van der Veen F., Mol B.W. 2005. IUI in male subfertility: Are we able to select the proper patients? *Reprod Biomed Online.* 11:624–31.
7. Steures P., Van der Steeg J.W., Hompes P.G., Bossuyt P.M., Habbema J.D., Eijkemans M.J. et al. 2007. Effectiveness of intrauterine insemination in subfertile couples with an isolated cervical factor: A randomized clinical trial. *Fertil Steril.* 88:1692–6.
8. Coppus S.F., Verhoeve H.R., Opmeer B.C., Van der Steeg J.W., Steures P., Eijkemans M.J., Hompes P.G., Bossuyt P.M., Van der Veen F., Mol B.W. 2007. Identifying subfertile ovulatory women for timely tubal patency testing: A clinical decision rule based on medical history. *Hum Reprod.* 22(10):2685–92.
9. de Wilde R.L. and Brosens I. 2012. Rationale of first-line endoscopy-based fertility exploration using transvaginal hydrolaparoscopy and minihysteroscopy. *Hum Reprod.* 27(8):2247–53.
10. Broeze K.A., Opmeer B.C., Coppus S.F., Van Geloven N., Den Hartog J.E., Land J.A., Van der Linden P.J.Q., Ng E.H.Y., Van der Steeg J.W., Steures P., Van der Veen F., and Mol B.W. 2012. Integration of patient characteristics and the results of chlamydia antibody testing and hysterosalpingography in the diagnosis of tubal pathology: An individual patient data meta-analysis. *Human Reprod.* 27: 2979–90.
11. Verhoeve H.R., Moolenaar L.M., Hompes P., Van der Veen F., and Mol B.W. 2012. Cost-effectiveness of tubal patency tests. *BJOG* October, accepted.

3

When to Start IUI?

Pieternel Steures and Jan Willem van der Steeg

Introduction

Subfertility has major socioeconomic consequences and a huge emotional impact on couples. Although many couples may already experience stress in the first year they are trying to conceive, basic fertility work-up is started after one year of unprotected intercourse without conception in case of an uneventful medical history (Chapter 2). In 5% of couples attending a gynecologist after one year of unprotected intercourse without conception a cervical factor is diagnosed, in 35% of couples mild male subfertility, in 5%, severe male subfertility, and in 35%, there is another reason for their subfertility. In 20% of couples no explanation for their subfertility is found.

In couples with cervical factor subfertility, male subfertility and unexplained subfertility intra-uterine insemination (IUI) is often the first step in the treatment cascade. IUI is easy to perform, inexpensive, and a minor burden to the couples. For these reasons, it is probably the most frequently performed treatment in daily fertility practice. In an IUI cycle, semen is processed in the laboratory and the motile spermatozoa are concentrated in a small volume. This is inseminated directly into the uterine cavity. Thus, the quintessence of IUI is based on three steps. First, semen processing based on the theory that by this process, the number of motile sperm is increased at the site of fertilization. Second, bypassing the possibly *hostile* cervical mucus and bringing the semen in closer proximity of the oocyt. Third, optimizing the timing by monitoring or inducing ovulation. All these steps should theoretically increase the probability of conception, especially in case of compromised semen parameters and cervical hostility. IUI can be performed with or without ovarian hyperstimulation. The aim of ovarian hyperstimulation is to correct subtle cycle disorders, to increase the number of available oocytes for fertilization, and to improve the timing of insemination.

Each assisted reproductive therapy with hyperstimulation of the ovaries carries risks and costs, and is a burden to the couple, therefore it is important to evaluate the effectiveness of treatment.

This chapter addresses the decision making of starting IUI by taking into account the prognosis and patient's preferences.

History

The first publication of a randomized clinical trial of IUI was in 1984 by Kerin et al. This trial included men with poor semen quality and compared the effectiveness of IUI on the day of the luteinizing hormone surge with intercourse in which timing was based on the basal body temperature and to intercourse in which timing was based on the luteinizing hormone surge. IUI was significantly more successful than the two other treatment policies. Since then, many randomized clinical trials that addressed the effectiveness of IUI were performed.

Until recently, the main emphasis in reproductive medicine has been on finding causal diagnoses for the couples' subfertility and to treat accordingly. In couples classified with unexplained subfertility, mild male subfertility, cervical factor subfertility, mild endometriosis, or one-sided tubal pathology, such a strict causal diagnosis has not been found and in these couples IUI is often considered.

However, IUI should only be offered to a couple if the success rate after IUI clearly exceeds the probability of a treatment independent pregnancy in that couple. Therefore, the prognosis should be taken into account in clinical decision making.

Prognostic Models

To be able to make adequate and reliable predictions in clinical practice, formal prediction models, in which the contribution of each factor is quantified, were developed in the recent past.

At the moment there are nine prediction models for spontaneous pregnancy, but only one model has been validated in an external population.[1] This is an extremely important issue, because most prediction models tend to be overoptimistic when applied to other populations than the one in which they were developed. This validated prediction model predicts accurately the chances of a treatment independent pregnancy among subfertile ovulatory couples. The prognostic variables in this model are female age, duration of subfertility, obstetric history, referral by general practitioner or another gynecologist and percentage progressive motile sperm. This model can be used by computer with the following URL: http://www.freya.nl/probability.php or with a paper score chart (Table 3.3 and Figure 3.1). If the model predicts a low treatment independent pregnancy chance, IUI can be considered.

By calculating the chance of an ongoing pregnancy after IUI, benefit from IUI in comparison to expectant management can be determined. There is one IUI prediction model that has been validated externally and has shown to be accurate.[2] The prognostic variables in this model are female age, duration of subfertility, diagnosis (cervical factor, male factor, or subfertility being unexplained), pathology (tubal, uterine, or endometriosis), the use and kind of ovarian hyperstimulation, and cycle number (Table 3.4 and Figure 3.2).

By using these models and comparing the prognoses generated by the models for the couple, they can be counseled on an individual basis. Such an approach can prevent overtreatment, decreases the misuse of facilities and other resources, and minimizes the risk of multiple pregnancy, which can be avoided by an expectant management.

Prognosis and Starting IUI

However, there are many trials on the effectiveness of IUI, randomized clinical trials that included the prognosis of the couple are scarce.

In couples with unexplained subfertility, 14 randomized studies are performed and included in a *Cochrane Review*.[3] These studies compared IUI with or without ovarian hyperstimulation with timed intercourse (TI), with or without ovarian hyperstimulation, IUI without controlled ovarian hyperstimulation to IUI with ovarian hyperstimulation, and IUI with *in vitro* fertilization (IVF).

Of these 14 studies, only three studies compared IUI with or without ovarian hyperstimulation to timed intercourse (without ovarian hyperstimulation) or expectant management. One of these studies took the prognosis into account. Nevertheless, the prognostic factors of the included couples in the three studies comparing IUI to timed intercourse or expectant management, seems to be comparable.[3] In these studies couples with an intermediate prognosis between 30 and 40% chance of an ongoing pregnancy resulting in a live born child in the next year were included. IUI without ovarian hyperstimulation was associated with higher ongoing pregnancy rates than expectant management, but these effects were not statistically significant, with an odds ratio (OR) of 1.5, 95% confidence interval (CI) 0.88 to 2.64. IUI with ovarian hyperstimulation offered no benefit over expectant management (OR ongoing pregnancy rate 1.0, 95% CI 0.67 to 1.5).

In couples with a cervical factor subfertility, six randomized studies were performed and discussed in a *Cochrane Review*.[4] Although these studies were all comparing IUI without ovarian hyperstimulation to timed intercourse or expectant management, the quality of five of the six trials was rather poor and

TABLE 3.3

Prediction Model for Spontaneous Pregnancy within 12 Months Leading to Live Birth (The formula for prediction of a spontaneous ongoing pregnancy is as follows: Pregnancy = $1-0.17 \times e((AGE\ 1 \times \beta1) + (AGE\ 2 \times \beta2) + (DUR \times \beta3) + (PRIM \times \beta4) + (PROG \times \beta5) + (REF \times \beta6))$.)

Variable	Regression Coefficient (β)	Category	Score Chart Index
Intercept	0.17	21–25	0
Maternal age if ≤31 years (per year older) (AGE 1)	−0.03 ($\beta1$)	26–31	2
Maternal age if >31 years (per year older than 31) (AGE 2)	−0.08 ($\beta2$)	32–35	6
		36–37	9
		38–39	11
		40–41	12
Duration of subfertility (per year longer) (DUR)	−0.19 ($\beta3$)	1	0
		2	2
		3–4	5
		5–6	9
		7–8	13
Primary subfertility of the couples (primary = 1, secondary = 0) (PRIM)	−0.58 ($\beta4$)	Primary	0
		Secondary	6
Progressive motile semen (%)[a] (PROG)	0.008 ($\beta5$)	≥60	0
		40–59	2
		20–39	4
		0–19	6
Referral status (tertiary couple = 1, secondary couple = 0)	−0.25 ($\beta6$)	Secondary	0
(REF)		Tertiary-care	4
		Sum	

Source: Hunault et al., 2004, *Human Reproduction*, with permission.

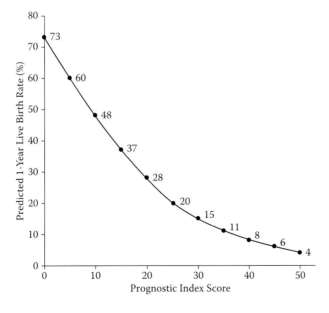

FIGURE 3.1 Prognostic Score Chart (From Hunault et al., *Human Reproduction,* 2004. With permission.) Example: A couple, with a 32-year-old woman, with primary subfertility of 1-year duration, with 20% progressive motile sperm, referred by the general practitioner has a prognostic index score of: 6 + 0 + 0 + 4 + 0 = 10, corresponding with a predicted 1-year live birth rate of 48%.

TABLE 3.4

Prognostic Score Chart for the Chance of an Ongoing Pregnancy after IUI (From Custers et al., *Fertil Steril*, 2007. With permission.)

						Prognostic Score
Female age	20 to 25	26 to 31	32 to 35	36 to 39	40 to 43	
Score	7	9	10	11	12	–
Dutation of subfertility	1 to 2	2 to 3	3 to 5	5 to 7	7 to 13	
Score	0	1	1	2	3	—
Diagnosis	Unexplained	Cervical factor	Male factor			
Score	0	–3	1			–
Pathology	Tubal	Uterine	Endometriosis			
Score	2	10	3			–
Ovarian hyperstimulation	No	CC	hMG or FSH			
Score	0	–2	–2			—
Cycle number	1	2	3	4	5 to 13	
Score	1	2	3	4	5	—
				Prognostic Index (sum score)		–

Circle the prognostic score for each of the variables and add them to the prognostic index. Use the curve in Figure 3.2 to estimate the chance of an ongoing pregnancy after the IUI treatment cycle.

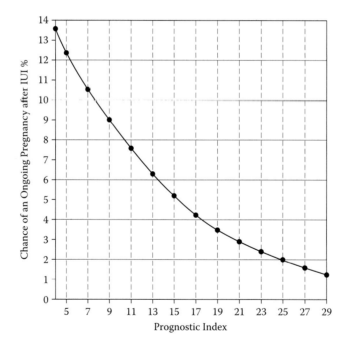

FIGURE 3.2 Prognostic index versus the chance of an ongoing pregnancy after IUI. (Example: A 33-year-old woman, with 2.5 years of unexplained subfertility, with no further pathology, and who will be treated with FSH has a prognostic index in the first cycle of: 10+1+0+0+–2+1=10. This score corresponds with 8.5% chance in the first treatment cycle). The prognostic index is calculated from the score chart in Table 3.4. The formula for prediction of an ongoing pregnancy after IUI is as follows: Probability=1/[1+exp(–β)] where β= –1.41 + (maternal age × –0.03) + duration of subfertility × –0.03) + (cervical factor × 0.27) + (male factor × –0.14) + (one-sided tubal pathology × –0.15) + (uterine anomaly × –0.98) + (endometriosis × –0.34) + (use of clomiphene citrate × 0.21) + (use of HMG or FSH × 0.23) + (cycle number (up to six) × –0.09).

due to the differences in participant characteristics and inconsistent clinical approaches to IUI, pooling of the results was not possible. In the only study that was taking the prognosis into account (being more than 30%), IUI was associated with higher ongoing pregnancy rates, albeit not statistically significant (relative risk: 1.6, 95% CI 0.91 to 2.8).

In couples with male factor subfertility, 20 randomized studies were performed, of which eight were eligible for the meta-analysis of the *Cochrane Review*.[5] Of these eight studies only one study compared IUI without ovarian hyperstimulation to timed intercourse (without ovarian hyperstimulation). For the comparison, IUI with ovarian hyperstimulation versus timed intercourse (without ovarian hyperstimulation) or expectant management no studies were found. In the only study to the effectiveness of IUI without ovarian hyperstimulation, IUI was five times more effective than timed intercourse. However, due to the small numbers (n = 21), the confidence interval is very wide (OR 5.29, 95% CI 0.42 to 66).

Patients' Preferences for IUI

Nowadays, patients' preferences are incorporated into medical decision making. The preferences of couples suffering from subfertility for IUI compared to expectant management and to IVF has been investigated in interviews.[6] In the interviews that compared IUI to expectant management, couples were offered scenarios in which the chance of a treatment independent pregnancy was varied against a fixed pregnancy chance after IUI with or without ovarian hyperstimulation. The results showed that even when the treatment independent pregnancy chances are still reasonable, couples prefer IUI with or without ovarian hyperstimulation to expectant management (probability of a treatment independent pregnancy 41 and 51% or lower, respectively). The risk of a multiple pregnancy did not affect patients' preferences. Instead, 77% of the couples continued IUI with ovarian hyperstimulation even at a 100% certainty of having a multiple pregnancy.

For the preferences of IUI compared to IVF, the majority of couples prefer continuation of IUI over IVF before they start IUI and after three cycles of IUI. After six cycles the preferences shift toward IVF.

Prognoses and IUI in Daily Practice

IUI with OH has not been shown to be effective in couples with cervical factor subfertility and unexplained subfertility and a good prognosis.[7] Therefore, the prognosis of the couples should be taken into account in clinical decision making. This enables us to distinguish those couples who may benefit from treatment from those who are unlikely to. Couples with an intermediate to good prognosis of a treatment independent pregnancy may be encouraged for expectant management and to postpone IUI for a while.

Since there are prognostic models and fertility registers, the use of prognostic models is easily accessible. It is of major importance to explain this to the couple at their first visit the prognostic approach. They have to know that if no causal diagnosis is found, their prognostic profile is being calculated and based on this prognosis, the best treatment policy will be determined.

However, it is essential to identify those couples that will benefit from IUI and those that will not, the exact cut-off point for the prognosis to treat or not to treat has not been assessed in a randomized clinical trial. In the existing trials 30% chance of a treatment independent pregnancy resulting in a live born child in the next year has been taken as the cut-off point. In the group with male subfertility there are still no studies with a prognostic approach. Therefore, randomized clinical trials on the effectiveness of IUI in couples with a poor prognosis or male subfertility are needed.

A second option might be to evaluate the existing studies at the patient level in an individual patient data (IPD) meta-analysis. By doing so the prognosis of the couples is extracted and automatically taken into account by the evaluation of the effectiveness of IUI.[8]

This study did not take the prognosis into account (Tables 3.1 and 3.2).

TABLE 3.1

Statements of Chapter 3

Statement	Level of Evidence (LOE)
In couples with a relatively good prognosis (>30%) of a treatment independent pregnancy, IUI should be postponed for at least 6 months	1b

TABLE 3.2

Recommendations of Chapter 3

Recommendation	Grade Strength
The prognosis of the couple should be taken into account in clinical decision making	A
The prognosis of the couple should be taken into account in the design of a randomized clinical trial	A

REFERENCES

1. Van der Steeg J.W., Steures P., Eijkemans M.J.C., Habbema J.D.F., Hompes P.G.A., Broekmans F.J., Van Dessel H.J.H.M., Bossuyt P.M.M., Van der Veen F., and Mol B.W.J. 2007. Pregnancy is predictable: A large-scale prospective external validation of the prediction of spontaneous pregnancy in subfertile couples. *Hum Reprod* 22:536–542.
2. Custers I.M., Steures P., Van der Steeg J.W., Van Dessel H.J.H.M., Bernardus R.E., Bourdrez P., Koks C.A., Riedijk W.J., Burggraaff J.M., Van der Veen F., and Mol B.W.J. 2007. External validation of a prediction model for an ongoing pregnancy after intrauterine insemination. *Fertil Steril* 88:425–431.
3. Verhulst S.M., Cohlen B.J., Hughes E., te Velde E., and Heineman M.J. 2011. Intra-uterine insemination for unexplained subfertility (review). *Cochrane Database Syst Rev* CD001838.
4. Helmerhorst F.M., Van Vliet H.A.A.M., Gornas T., Finken M.J., and Grimes D.A. 2010. Intra-uterine insemination versus timed intercourse or expectant management for cervical hostility in subfertile couples (review). *Cochrane Database Syst Rev* CD002809.
5. Bensdorp A., Cohlen B.J., Heineman M.J., and Vanderkerchove P. 2010. Intra-uterine insemination for male subfertility (review). *Cochrane Database Syst Rev* CD000360.
6. Steures P., Berkhout J.C., Hompes P.G.A., Van der Steeg J.W., Bossuyt P.M.M., Van der Veen F., Habbema J.D.F., Eijkemans M.J.C., and Mol B.W.J. 2005. Patients' preferences in deciding between intrauterine insemination and expectant management. *Hum Reprod* 20:752–755.
7. Steures P., Van der Steeg J.W., Hompes P.G., Habbema J.D., Eijkemans M.J., Broekmans F.J. et al. 2006. Intrauterine insemination with controlled ovarian hyperstimulation versus expectant management for couples with unexplained subfertility and an intermediate prognosis: A randomised clinical trial. *Lancet* 368(9531):216–221.
8. Janes H. and Pepe M.S. 2008. Adjusting for covariates in studies of diagnostic, screening, or prognostic markers: An old concept in a new setting. *Am J Epidemiol* 168:89–97.
9. Hunault et al. 2004. Two new prediction rules for spontaneous pregnancy leading to live birth among subfertile couples, based on the synthesis of three previous models. *Hum Reprod* 19(9):2019–2026.

4

Indications for IUI

Ben Cohlen and Hasan N. Sallam

Introduction

Intra-uterine insemination (IUI) is an ancient technique already reported in 1790. In the early days the ejaculate of the husband was inseminated without preparation resulting in uterine cramps and increasing the probability of tubal infections. With the arrival of IVF, semen preparation techniques were developed and IUI regained its popularity, being more safe and painless. The rationale behind IUI is increasing the number of motile sperm that are morphologically normal at the site of fertilization. Bypassing the cervix, which acts as a reservoir for sperm, increases the importance of adequate timing of the insemination (see Chapter 14).

At this moment IUI is probably one of the most applied assisted reproductive techniques worldwide. Nevertheless, there is still an ongoing debate whether or not IUI is an effective treatment option for various indications.

To (dis)prove a beneficial effect of IUI this technique should be compared with expected management in a well-described population in a large (multi-center) randomized trial. In many of these (older) trials expectant management was often "replaced" by timed intercourse. *Cochrane Reviews* have been published on this subject[1–3] and will provide a (solid) basis for this chapter.

Overview of Existing Evidence

The following indications are often mentioned with regard to IUI with partner's sperm:

- Cervical factor
- Male subfertility
- Unexplained subfertility
- Endometriosis
- Sexual disorders
- Ovarian dysfunction

In case of an isolated cervical factor, defined as a repeated negative postcoital test despite adequate timing and normal sperm parameters, IUI in natural cycles significantly increases the probability of conception (LOE 1b).[4] A debate is ongoing whether or not postcoital testing should be part of a routine fertility work-up. It has been shown that in case of a cervical factor adding ovarian hyperstimulation does not improve pregnancy rates (LOE 2).

When a male factor is present the latest *Cochrane Review* clearly states that there is insufficient evidence to conclude whether IUI is effective or not (LOE 1a).[1] Older evidence, often from crossover trials and expressed as pregnancy rate per completed cycle, found a significant beneficial effect of IUI. Nowadays results should be expressed as live birth rates (or at least ongoing pregnancy rates) per couple applying intention to treat analysis. From crossover trials the results of the first cycle only can be used in meta-analyses. Nevertheless, the evidence from older trials do point out that there might be a place for IUI in case of a moderate male factor.

The total number of motile sperm inseminated has the ability to predict failure: in other words, when less than 0.8–5 million motile sperm are inseminated, pregnancies hardly occur (LOE 1a).[5] This wide spread in lower cut-off levels indicates that large differences exist between hospitals. It is advised that each clinic defines its own cut-off level of success. Most clinics apply cut-off levels of 0.8–1.0 million.

When the total motile sperm count before sperm preparation has an average value above 10 million, almost resembling couples with unexplained subfertility, mild ovarian hyperstimulation (MOH) might be added (LOE 1b). Some clinics will consider these couples unexplained, others would still call it (mild) male subfertility. Immunologic male infertility is discussed in Chapter 4.

IUI in natural cycles has no significant beneficial effect over expectant management when the subfertility of the couple is unexplained (LOE 1a).[3] This conclusion has been confirmed in a large multi-center trial (LOE 1b). This trial found no effect of clomiphene citrate combined with unrestricted intercourse in couples with unexplained subfertility either. It has been proven, however, that the combination of ovarian hyperstimulation and IUI significantly improves live birth rates in these couples (LOE 1a).[3] This conclusion is based on a meta-analysis of various trials in which rather aggressive stimulation has been applied in some of them, resulting in high multiple pregnancy rates. Whether the addition of mild ovarian hyperstimulation, resulting in 2 to 3 dominant follicles only, significantly improves live birth rates has not been proven yet.

In patients with endometriosis American Fertility Society (AFS) grade 1 or 2, the exact mechanism of declined fertility remains unanswered. When adhesions are present one can understand a declined pick-up mechanism but when small spots of endometriosis are present only, an explanation is more difficult to give. It has been assumed that in case of mild endometriosis, couples should be treated as couples with unexplained subfertility and patients might benefit from IUI in combination with MOH (LOE 1b). On the other hand, there is evidence that during laparoscopy ablation of endometriotic lesions plus adhesiolysis is effective in enhancing spontaneous pregnancy compared to diagnostic laparoscopy alone (LOE 1a). There seems no role for IUI with or without ovarian stimulation in moderate to severe endometriosis.

In case of physiological and psychological sexual dysfunction, such as hypospadias, vaginismus, retrograde ejaculation, and impotence, there is often no need for IUI, as semen might be placed intra-vaginal or intra-cervical. When semen parameters are low, as often is the case in men with retrograde ejaculation, semen preparation is mandatory followed by IUI.

In literature, IUI is often applied in couples with *ovarian dysfunction* as well. In women with anovulation, ovulation induction should be the treatment of first choice. When the male partner has sufficient motile sperm, ovulation induction can be combined with unrestricted intercourse and the addition of IUI has not been proven effective. Ovulation induction should result in mono-follicular development and mono-ovulation whereas MOH used in combination with IUI strives for multi-follicular development and the release of two to three oocytes (LOE 1a).

Discussion

IUI is still an assisted reproductive technology under debate. On the one hand, it has been shown that treatment with IUI should not be started too soon (Chapter 3) as spontaneous chances of pregnancy might still be favorable in couples with male or unexplained subfertility (higher than 30–40%). On the other hand, IVF and ICSI are becoming more and more cost-effective and safe. Nevertheless, it has been shown that IUI can improve conception rates significantly and it therefore deserves a place in the armamentarium of reproductive technologies. IUI is a relatively simple, noninvasive, cheap option for couples with patent tubes and a sufficient number of motile sperm after semen preparation. When offered, three to nine cycles of IUI can result in cumulative pregnancy rates of 25 to 50% and many couples can be prevented from moving on to IVF. In countries where society is willing to invest in reproductive treatments, IUI with or without MOH should be offered before starting more invasive treatment options like IVF. Couples should not be forced to choose between these options. In developing countries with restricted resources IUI is often the only option. It is very important that IUI is applied for the right indications, not too early and in a safe and controlled manner.

Conclusions

It is concluded that IUI in natural cycles should be applied in couples with a proven cervical factor, and it can be applied in couples with a moderate male factor defined as less than on average 10 million motile sperm in the ejaculate but more than 800,000 motile sperm after preparation. IUI with MOH should be offered to couples with unexplained subfertility, mild endometriosis, and a mild male factor (see also Tables 4.1 and 4.2).

TABLE 4.1

Statements of Chapter 4

Statement	Level of Evidence (LOE)
In couples with a cervical factor subfertility, IUI in natural cycles significantly increases the probability of conception	1b
In couples with a relatively good prognosis for spontaneous pregnancy, IUI should not be applied too soon	1b
The total number of motile sperm inseminated has the ability to predict failure: in other words, when less than 0.8–5 million motile sperm are inseminated, pregnancies hardly occur	1a
When a male factor is present, there is insufficient evidence to conclude whether IUI is effective or not	1a
IUI in natural cycles has no significant beneficial effect over expectant management when the subfertility of the couple is unexplained	1a
In couples with unexplained subfertility, the combination of ovarian hyperstimulation and IUI significantly improves live birth rates	1a
When the total motile sperm count before sperm preparation has an average value above 10 million, defined as a mild male factor, mild ovarian hyperstimulation might be added	1b
In case of mild endometriosis (AFS grade 1 or 2) couples should be treated as couples with unexplained subfertility and patients might benefit from IUI in combination with mild ovarian hyperstimulation	1b
Mild ovarian hyperstimulation for IUI should result in the release of 2 to 3 oocytes	1a

TABLE 4.2

Recommendations of Chapter 4

Recommendation	Grade Strength
In couples with a relatively good prognosis for spontaneous conception, IUI should not be started too soon	A
In couples with mild male subfertility with an average TMSC of $\geq$ 10 million, ovarian hyperstimulation should be added	A
IUI should not be applied when less than 0.8–5.0 million motile sperm are present after semen preparation	A
IUI can be applied in natural cycles in case of cervical hostility and probably in case of a moderate male subfertility	A
In couples with unexplained subfertility or mild endometriosis receiving IUI, ovarian hyperstimulation should be added. IUI in natural cycles should not be applied in these couples	A

REFERENCES

1. Bensdorp A.J., Cohlen B.J., Heineman M.J., and Vandekerckhove P. 2007. Intra-uterine insemination for male subfertility. *Cochrane Database Syst Rev* (4):CD000360.
2. Cantineau A.E., Cohlen B.J., and Heineman M.J. 2007. Ovarian stimulation protocols (anti-oestrogens, gonadotrophins with and without GnRH agonists/antagonists) for intrauterine insemination (IUI) in women with subfertility. *Cochrane Database Syst Rev* (2):CD005356.
3. Verhulst S.M., Cohlen B.J., Hughes E., te Velde E., and Heineman MJ. 2006. Intra-uterine insemination for unexplained subfertility. *Cochrane Database Syst Rev* (4):CD001838.
4. Steures P., Van der Steeg J.W., Hompes P.G., Bossuyt P.M., Habbema J.D., Eijkemans M.J., Schols W.A., Burggraaff J.M., Van der Veen F., and Mol B.W. 2007. Effectiveness of intrauterine insemination in subfertile couples with an isolated cervical factor: A randomized clinical trial. *Fertil Steril* 88(6):1692–1696.
5. Van Weert J.M., Repping S., Van Voorhis B.J., Van der Veen F., Bossuyt P.M., and Mol B.W. 2004. Performance of the postwash total motile sperm count as a predictor of pregnancy at the time of intra-uterine insemination: A meta-analysis. *Fertil Steril* 82(3):612–620.

5

Immunologic Male Infertility

Benny Verheyden

Immunologic male infertility is considered an important issue among fertility specialists. The problem is recognized as difficult to treat, and the results of intra-uterine insemination (IUI) programs are stated to be poor. Several statements are considered true, but a regard of evidence-based data shows that they are scarce and hard to find. The belief among peers shows this is not proved in any evidence-based way.

The Origin of Immunologic Male Infertility

For more than a century, the antigenic capacity of sperm has been known. Several experiments have shown that subcutaneous injection of one's own sperm can provoke an allergic reaction on the skin showing a red and itching papula. Rümke and Wilson demonstrated in 1954 that the occurrence of antisperm antibodies (ASAs) in male subjects is associated with infertility. Since that time it has been accepted that an immunological response against spermatozoa—humoral or cellular—can be a cause of infertility.

The origin of immunologic infertility seems to be clear. During fetal development, at the end of the third trimester, the immune system establishes tolerance to all self-antigens. At that time, no spermatozoa are present. The fetal testis only contains spermatogonial stem cells, Sertoli cells, and Leydig cells, which are all diploid. These cells (except the Leydig cells) are quiescent, that is, not producing any protein, not even showing any metabolism at that time. From puberty onward, long after the *immunologic auto scan* has been finished, spermatogenesis starts up, producing quadriploid and haploid cells, and synthesizing several proteins important for procreation, although not recognized by the immune system as *proper to the own body*. This is the cornerstone for male immunologic infertility.

All elements of spermatogenesis are *strange to the immune system* and have to be isolated from the immune system at once. Several mechanisms are able to do so. The first and most important mechanism is the tight junctions between the Sertoli cells. They represent the blood testis barrier separating the maturing sperm cells from the bloodstream. Once the spermatogonial stem cell starts developing, it passes through the gap junction into an environment of *immunologic silence*. Inside the tubulus, no immunological cells (leukocytes, lymphocytes) are encountered. This means that no immunologic response to any protein can be evoked. Within the testis, this isolation is achieved rather completely by the blood-testis barrier. In other parts of the genital tract, the epithelial lining, supplemented by other local immunosuppressive barriers, can be responsible for this isolation.

Tung[1] postulated that small amounts of spermatozoal antigens continuously leak into the genital tubules of the epididymis and the vas, activating suppressor T lymphocytes, which inhibit the immune response. This multi-focal system completes the immune inhibition, preventing the generation of ASAs under normal circumstances.

Clinical Situations Provoking the Generation of Antisperm Antibodies

In developed countries the most important origin of ASAs is probably vasectomy. More than 80% of vasectomized males develop ASAs during the first year following their operation. In most cases it concerns IgGs, which are considered to be less harmful. Nevertheless, even IgAs are frequently found in these males, considering that this type of ASA interferes more powerfully with fertility. Immunological infertility can, however, be brought about by several other clinical situations as torsion of the testis, varicocele, testicular trauma, and orchitis.

Sharp trauma to the testicle, as a testicular biopsy, is mostly a safe procedure, not provoking ASAs. Blunt testicular trauma, however, gives rise to risk for the development of ASAs. Nevertheless, much controversy exists over the clinical relevance of sperm auto-antibodies. Although many antibodies have been found in seminal fluid and antigen–antibody complexes have been found in sperm, the direct effect of these antigen–antibody interactions are still not known.

Moreover, until now, no study has characterized the type and titer that causes infertility.

How to Detect Antisperm Antibodies (ASAs)

Independent of the characteristics of the spermatozoa, that is, concentration, motility, and morphology, the presence of ASAs on the motile sperm cells will induce the diagnosis of an immunologic cause. An immunologic evaluation is recommended when (1) semen analysis shows aggregates of sperm, (2) although other sperm parameters are normal, extreme asthenozoöspermia is seen with normal vitality, (3) there is a clinical risk for immunological infertility, and (4) there is an unexplained infertility with a normal semen analysis.

In practice, four types of tests can be used to detect and to quantify antisperm antibodies.

> *Agglutination Tests* detect the presence of ASAs on the surface antigens of the spermatozoa by their ability to cause agglutination. The reference test is the tray agglutination test (TAT).[2]
>
> Specificity of this test is, however, lowered by the fact that a nonimmunological factor can cause agglutination, as the presence of bacteria, fungi, or amorphous material in the seminal plasma. Therefore, the test can be used as a first screening, but it has to be confirmed by other more specific tests.
>
> *Complement Dependent Tests* detect antibodies reacting with antigens on the sperm cell membrane due to their cytotoxic effect. Best known is the sperm immobilization test.[3] The test is very specific, but only detects IgG antibodies and not the IgAs, which are more important for male immunologic infertility.
>
> *Enzyme-Linked Immunosorbant Assays* are more expensive, less sensitive, and more time consuming, and therefore less frequently used.
>
> *Immunoglobulin Binding Tests* can detect the presence of antibodies on spermatozoa by means of antibodies directed against human immunoglobulins. These antiglobulins can be labeled or bound to indicator cells or particles. Labels used can be fluorescence molecules, radio-isotopes, or enzymes. Particles used are red blood cells, latex particles, or polyacrilamide beads.

The most popular tests used in the basic semen analysis lab (BSA lab) are the MAR test (mixed antiglobulin reaction) and the immunobead test. These tests are easy to perform, robust, and cheap. The direct mixed antiglobulin test (direct MAR) was first described by Jager in 1978 to detect ASAs bound to sperm cells in fresh semen. As indicator cells, immunoglobulin coated red blood cells were initially used, and agglutination of the red blood cells with motile spermatozoa in the presence of antiglobulin were studied. If more than 50% of the sperm cells were covered with red blood cells, the fertility problem could be considered as immunological. Also, information about the location of the ASAs on the sperm cells could be provided.

Until now, the sperm MAR has continuously been improved. Red blood cells are replaced by latex particles, making the test more practical and sensitive. Initially, only the IgG class of antibodies could be detected; at the moment testing for (the more important) IgA class is available. The test can also be performed indirectly to detect ASAs in serum and seminal plasma, and there seems to be a good correlation between direct test results in fresh semen and indirect test results in seminal plasma and serum.[4]

The immunobead test was developed by Clarke in 1985. This test uses polyacrylamide beads coated with antibodies against human IgG, IgM, and IgA. This test is also robust, but more time consuming since it requires washing the sperm several times in order to remove the seminal plasma. This test also can be performed directly using motile sperm cells, or indirectly using serum or seminal plasma.

How ASAs Interfere with Fertility

The most obvious way ASAs are responsible for male infertility is by agglutination of the sperm cells after ejaculation. This results in lowering of their motility and their ability to penetrate the cervical mucus. If more than 50% of sperm are bound to antibodies, reduced cervical mucus penetration can result. This occurs because the Fc regions of the immunoglobulins are interacting with receptors on the cervical mucus. In particular, IgA antibodies are mediating this phenomenon, making them more harmful for fertilization than IgGs.

There are, however, more mechanisms by which ASAs are interfering with conception. These mechanisms can be grouped into disturbances of sperm transport and disruptions in gamete interaction. After passing the cervical mucous barrier, ASAs can induce phagocytotic cleaning of the sperm cells by macrophages or inhibit sperm capacitation or acrosome reaction. Also, zona binding and penetration, and oölemma binding can be influenced. It has been described that even ASAs can impair pronucleus formation. Several recent papers make it clear that immunologic male infertility acts not only on the motility of sperm cells.

Management of Immunologic Male Infertility

The results of causal treatment of immunologic male infertility by corticosteroids were published by several authors in the 19th century. The results expressed as an improvement in pregnancy rates were very poor. Complications, however, are high. Side effects such as bone demineralization occur in up to 60% of the patients, some of them resulting in fractures or aseptic necrosis of the femoral head. Also, diabetes can be induced by high doses of corticoids. Moreover, this therapy seemed to be effective in patients with low number of sperm cells agglutinating in the MAR tests.

In Utero Insemination (IUI) for Immunologic Male Infertility

The choice of the most appropriate assisted reproductive treatment for the individual couple is often a difficult one.[5] This is even more than obvious in couples with immunologic male infertility, especially in couples after a refertilization procedure after vasectomy. Although it is widely accepted that in severe cases of immunologic male infertility, where most of the spermatozoa, that is, >80%, are antibody coated, ICSI has to be recommended; IUI can play a particular role in the treatment of this situation. Ombelet et al.[6] showed in a crossover study that IUI can be a first choice treatment in patients with immunologic infertility. Four cycles of IUI (with or without ovulatory stimulation) can be offered before proceeding to an IVF program.

Andrologists and fertility specialists aim to offer patients the least invasive procedure in fulfilling their birth wish. Moreover, this is also an important medico-economical issue. Therefore, there is a need for a good pretreatment tool predicting the success rate of in utero insemination in couples with immunologic male infertility. The postwash total motile concentration (pTMC) may have a unique value as a prognostic tool, since it reflects the motile sperm available for insemination. Nevertheless, no studies are available confirming this theory, not in the overall subfertile population, nor in the immunologic subgroup.

TABLE 5.1

Statements of Chapter 5

Statement	Level of Evidence (LOE)
In case of immunologic infertility, adding 2% albumine to the buffering medium upon sperm retrieval is useful	4
IUI is the first choice before proceeding to IVF/ICSI in case of immunologic infertility	2a

TABLE 5.2

Recommendations of Chapter 5

Recommendation	Grade Strength
It is advised to add 2% albumine to the buffering medium upon sperm retrieval in case of immunologic infertility	GPP
In case of immunologic infertility IUI should be offered before starting IVF/ICSI	B

The importance of teratozoospermia has however been shown: a clear drop in pregnancy rate has been reported when less than 4% ideal forms (strict criteria Tygerberg) are present.[5] Lahteenmaki[7] showed in a comparative crossover study that IUI resulted in higher pregnancy rates than low dose corticosteroids in males with immunologic infertility, without even taking into account the important adverse effects. An additional value surely is the sperm preparation technique.

In vitro treatment of the spermatozoa with chemotrypsin prior to IUI can increase the pregnancy rate.[8] Also, collecting the semen immediately in HTF medium with albumin can improve motility in the native sample as well as after sperm preparation, making the IUI possible.[9]

However, evidence-based studies, with a regard to the success rate of IUI in couples with immunologic male infertility, cannot be found. This particular group of patients is always making a part of *overall* trials, in studying the success of IUI. In general, the usefulness of IUI in male subfertility is still under debate[10]; the effectiveness of IUI in couples with ASAs is highly controversial.

Looking into the Future

Until now, little is known about the biochemical nature of the antigens inducing the production of ASAs. Tests look for a mixed antiglobulin reaction, without any more specificity. Nevertheless, it seems obvious that the impact on fertility of several ASAs is not the same. There is clearly a need for better differentiation of the different types of antibodies. This issue is not only important for treating immunologic infertility and especially infertility persisting despite vasovasostomy, but it can also open a new field of immunologic anticonception.

REFERENCES

1. Tung K.S.K. Autoimmunity of the testis. 1980. In Dhindsa D.S. and Schumacher G.F.B., eds. *Immunological Aspects of Infertility and Fertility Regulation*. New York: Elsevier North-Holland.
2. Friberg J. 1974. A simple and sensitive micromethod for demonstration of sperm-agglutinating activity in the semen from infertile men. *Acta Gynecol Scand* (Suppl)36:21.
3. Isojima S., Li T.S., and Ashitaka Y. 1968. Immunologic analysis of sperm mobilizing factor found in sera of women with unexplained infertility. *Am J Ostet Gynecol* 101:677.
4. Vermeulen A. and Comhaire F. 1983. Le test "MAR" aux particules de latex et le test spermatoxique selon Suominen: Simplification et nouveauté dans l'arsenal du diagnostic immunologique. *Contraception, Fertilité et Sexualité* 11:381–384.
5. Van Waert J., Kruger T.F., Lombard C.J., and Ombelet W. 2001. Predictive value of normal sperm morphology in intrauterine insemination: A structured literature review. *Hum Repr* (Update) 7(5):495–500.

6. Ombelet W. et al. 1997. Treatment of male infertility due to sperm surface antibodies: IUI or IVF? *Hum Reprod* 12(6):165–170.
7. Lähteenmäki A., Veilahti J., and Hovatta O. 1995. Intra-uterine insemination versus cyclic, low dose prednisolone in couples with male antisperm antibodies. *Hum Reprod* Jan. 10(1):142–147.
8. Check J.H., Hourani W., Check M.L., Graziano V., and Levin E. 2004. Effect of treating antibody-coated sperm with chymotrypsin on pregnancy rates following IUI as compared outcome to IVF/ICSI. *Arch Androl* 50(2):93–95.
9. Verheyden B. Unpublished data.
10. Bensdorp A.J., Cohlen B.J., Heineman M.J., and Vandekerckhove P. 2007. *Cochrane Database Syst Rev* Oct. (4).

ADVISED LITERATURE

Nieschlag E., Behre, H.M., and Nieschlag S. 2010. *Andrology, Male Reproductive Health and Dysfunction*, 3rd ed. Berlin: Springer.
Lipshultz L.J. and Howards S.S. 1996. *Infertility in the Male*, 3rd ed. St Louis: Mosby.
Mortimer D. 1994. *Practical Laboratory Andrology*. Oxford: Oxford University Press.

6

Factors Influencing IUI Outcome: Female Age

Felicia Yarde and Frank J.M. Broekmans

Reproductive Aging[1]

It has long been understood that reproductive success in the female is strongly associated with age. With increasing chronological age, female fecundity (the ability to produce viable offspring) decreases. This phenomenon is based on studies in historical populations, where no consistent contraceptive methods were used and on studies in women undergoing donor inseminations. These observations have shown the gradual decline in monthly fecundity rate after the age of 30 years. From 36 years onward this decline occurs more rapidly, with the end of natural fertility occurring, on average, as early as 41 years.

The human species can be considered as relatively infertile compared to many animal species, with a monthly fecundity rate of only 20%. This indicates that even healthy fertile couples would require many exposure months to conceive, with age-related decline in fecundity further extending the necessary time frame for natural conception. Therefore, the proportion of infertile couples in their 20s is only 4%, compared to 10–20% in women over 35 years. These infertility rates can increase up to 50% for moderately fecund women over 35 years, who have unsuccessfully tried to conceive for many years (Table 6.1).

Ovarian Aging[1]

Changes in ovarian function, dominated by the gradual decline of both oocyt quantity and quality, are major contributors to the reproductive aging process. The latter becomes apparent both in increasing rates of infertility observed at older age as well as increased aneuploidy rates, responsible for a higher risk of miscarriage and trisomic births with increasing age.

The size of a woman's follicle and oocyte stock is already determined during early stages of fetal development. At birth, this primordial follicle pool consists of around 1–2 million oocytes. Due to a continuous process of apoptosis, follicle numbers are reduced to approximately 300,000–400,000 at menarche. When follicle numbers fall below a critical threshold of a few thousand, the perimenopausal transition commences, which is characterized by overt cycle irregularity and altered cycle length. Finally, prolonged menstrual cycles proceed to cycle arrest, a milestone referred to as menopause, which coincides with a near absence of primordial follicles in the ovaries.

Figure 6.1 demonstrates a model for the gradual loss of primordial follicles through the stages of reproductive life of the female.

The normal process of ovarian aging varies considerably among women, with peak fertility in the mid- to late 20s. The profound age-related decline in female fecundity, however, remains largely unnoticed until clinical signs of the perimenopausal transition are present. The loss of the capacity to create an ongoing pregnancy leading to a live birth is accompanied by an increase in early follicular follicle-stimulating hormone (FSH) levels, which cannot be easily recognized by an individual. The onset of the menopausal transition, expressed by lengthened cycles due to deficiency of antral follicles capable of growing into dominance, is usually a woman's first notification of advanced ovarian aging. Figure 6.2 demonstrates the stages of reproductive aging.

Despite the individual variation in onset of menopause, a fixed time interval is believed to be present among the stages of reproductive aging. From natural population studies an apparent variation in the age

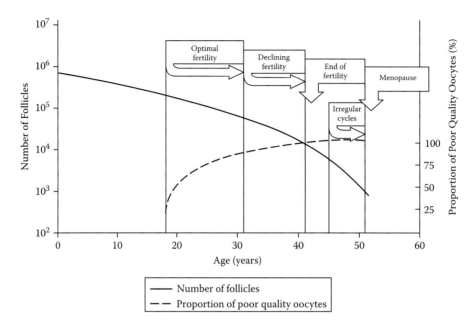

FIGURE 6.1   Schematic representation of the number of primordial follicles present in the ovaries and the chromocomal quality of oocytes in relation to female age and corresponding reproductive events. (Data derived from Hansen et al., 2008, *Hum Reprod,* March 23(3):699–708; de Bruin et al., 2001 *Hum Reprod,* September 16(9):2014–2018. Graph reproduced from Broekmans F.J., Soules M.R., and Fauser B.C., 2009, *Endocr Rev,* August 30(5):465–493, with permission from the Endocrine Society.)

at last childbirth between age 31 and 50 years has been observed, with a distribution shape highly similar to the one for menopause. The presumed fixed time interval between menopause and natural sterility may prove of great clinical importance to provide information concerning a woman's individual fertility life span. Early menopause suggests an early loss of natural fertility resulting in infertility at a young age, and vice versa.

Postponing Childbearing[1]

Since the introduction of steroid contraceptive methods in the 1960s, together with growing economic wealth, women gained opportunities to increase their education levels and participate in the labor force. As a result, age at first birth increased considerably by postponing first childbearing. Due to these trends, an increasing proportion of women will fail to conceive within a time frame of 12 months. This condition, referred to as infertility, is causing a growing proportion of couples to be dependent on assisted reproductive technology (ART), such as intra-uterine insemination (IUI), to conceive.

However, ART will only compensate for the decreased natural fertility to a limited extent, leaving many couples involuntarily childless.

Infertility[2]

A number of key events are essential for conception to occur. Next to ovulation, fallopian tube pick-up of the oocyte and fertilization, transport of the embryo through the fallopian tubes, and implantation of the embryo once having made contact with the endometrial surface, are necessary steps in the process of achieving an ongoing pregnancy.

Abnormalities in one or more steps of this process may result in infertility. Anovulation or oligo-ovulation accounts for approximately 20% of the infertility cases, with polycystic ovarian syndrome (PCOS) being the underlying cause in the vast majority of cases. Tubal factor infertility accounts for about 35% of all infertility cases.[2] However, it should be noted that the prevalence of tubal factor infertility differs strongly

Menarche						FMP (0)			

Stage	−5	−4	−3b	−3a	−2	−1	+1a	+1b	+1c	+2
Terminology	REPRODUCTIVE				MENOPAUSAL TRANSITION		POSTMENOPAUSE			
	Early	Peak	Late		Early	Late	Early			Late
					Perimenopause					
Duration	Variable				Variable	1–3 years	2 years (1+1)	3–6 years		*Remaining life span*
PRINCIPAL CRITERIA										
Menstrual Cycle	Variable to regular	Regular	Regular	Subtle changes in Flow's Length	*Variable Length* Persistent ≥7-day difference in length of Consecutive cycles	Interval of amenor-rhea of > = 60 days				
SUPPORTIVE CRITERIA										
Endocrine FSH AMH Inhibin B			Low Low	Variable* Low Low	↑Variable* Low Low	↑>25IU/L** Low Low	↑Variable Low Low	Stabilizes Very low Very low		
Antral Follicle Count			Low	Low	Low	Low	Very Low	Very Low		
DESCRIPTIVE CHARACTERISTICS										
Symptoms						Vasomotor symptoms *Likely*	Vasomotor symptoms *Most Likely*			*Increasing symptoms of urogenital atrophy*

* Blood draw on cycle days 2–5 ↑ = elevated.

** Approximate expected level based on assays using current international pituitary standard.

FIGURE 6.2 The stages of Reproductive Aging Workshop staging system demonstrates the relation between alterations in cycle regularity and endocrine changes across the various stages of reproductive aging. FMP = final menstrual period; FSH = follicle-stimulating hormone; AMH = antimüllerian hormone. (Reproduced from Harlow S., Executive Summary of the Stages of the Reproductive Aging Workshop et al., 2012, *Journal of Clinical Endocrinology & Metabolism*, 97; 1159–68, with permission from the Endocrine Society.)

between different countries and continents, with a prevalence of up to 80% in developing countries in sub-Saharan Africa. Next to female factors, a small proportion of infertility is caused by obvious male factors such as azoospermia and severe oligospermia. Mild male factor and unexplained infertility together with infertility associated with advancing female age accounts for 50–60% of all couples presenting with fertility problems. Specifically, for mild male factor and unexplained infertility, it may be stated that a real explanation seems absent. Therefore, treatment of these couples first relies on a simple mode of assisted conception: IUI with or without ovarian hyperstimulation (OH).

IUI[3]

Several prognostic factors for the outcome of IUI treatment have been identified and include female age, semen parameters, duration of infertility, and treatment characteristics. For this chapter, we will focus on female age and its effect on IUI outcome.

IUI and Female Age[1]

Around the globe, female age is a limiting factor for any kind of ART treatment. Age as a limiting factor for IUI success is based on the probability of achieving an ongoing pregnancy, which is reduced with increasing age to approximately zero after the mean age of 41 years. Specifically in unexplained and mild semen factor infertility, the effect of female age on the failure to conceive is suggested to be extensive. When applying IUI treatment, use is made of one or two oocytes that may have the same quality deficit as in the spontaneous situation. In addition, female fecundity may vary across women. This is why older women will be tested for their ovarian reserve status before getting access to treatment and women of 41 years onward are often denied treatment, even if quantitative ovarian reserve may still seem sufficient.

In addition, other issues may play a role in the decision-making process. An increased risk of pregnancy complications is observed in women over 40 years. Especially, preeclampsia, preterm birth, and perinatal death are complications, which seem to be clearly raised. In terms of cost-benefit and cost-effectiveness, no Level 1 studies have systemically analyzed at what age IUI becomes (cost-) nonbeneficial (Table 6.2).

Data on the effects of female age on the outcome of IUI is limited. To study these effects, most preferably we would conduct a study in women of any age undergoing IUI treatment with or without standard OH and observe the outcome of live births both per cycle started as well as per treatment period. In this ideal situation, no selection occurs based on female or reproductive age (ovarian reserve characteristics) and treatment approach is not affected by prior knowledge of age or ovarian reserve. Unfortunately, such studies, where both selection and verification bias have been prevented, are quite rare. In the following section we will summarize existing literature studying the effect of female age on IUI outcome for couples using husbands' sperm, IUI outcome with donor sperm, and the additional value of ovarian hyperstimulation.

IUI: Female Age and Husband's Sperm[4]

Based on the existing literature, we can conclude that female age is the most important factor influencing the likelihood of pregnancy in IUI with husband's sperm. The indication for IUI treatment, male factor, or unexplained infertility has no clear impact on prospects for pregnancy. Ongoing pregnancy rates per couple differed from 38.5% in women under the age of 30 years to 12.5% in women over 40 years. In addition, delivery rates after IUI treatment also revealed a sharp decline in women over the age of 40 years.

IUI: Female Age and Donor Sperm[4]

Even more limited is the data concerning the age effect on IUI with donor sperm. Based on three retrospective cohort studies, cumulative pregnancy rates clearly decreased with increasing female age. However, acceptable pregnancy rates have been reached up until the age of 42 years.

The overall delivery rate in IUI with donor sperm is 14% per cycle with an expected cumulative delivery rate of 77% after 12 IUI cycles. Subgroup analyses based on female age illustrated a decline in expected cumulative delivery rate after 12 cycles from 55% in 40-year-old women to 20% if aged 43 years. Figure 6.3 demonstrates the fecundity per IUI cycle with donor sperm according to female age.

IUI: Female Age and Mild Ovarian Stimulation[3]

IUI treatment can be combined with mild to moderate ovarian stimulation by the use of oral clomiphene citrate and/or exogenous gonadotrophins and/or sequential clomiphene citrate/gonadotrophins. A true benefit has only been demonstrated for the combination of IUI with OH in couples with unexplained infertility. Unfortunately, many studies did not take female age into account when studying the adjuvant role of OH to counteract the adverse age effect, leaving only a few limited quality studies.

From these studies it appears that OH in combination with IUI results in significantly higher pregnancy rates than natural cycle timed IUI alone. However, ovarian stimulation carries a risk of inducing multiple

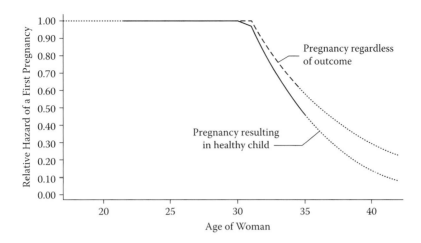

FIGURE 6.3 Fecundity per IUI cycle with donor sperm according to female age. Mean rate for women aged 20–30 was scaled at 1.00. For a woman aged 33 years, the relative rate of 0.75 indicates that she has in each IUI cycle 75% of the chance of a woman aged 20–30 years to become pregnant. (Reproduced from Broekmans F.J., Soules M.R., and Fauser B.C., 2009, *Endocr Rev*, August 30(5):465–93, with permission from the Endocrine Society.)

pregnancies. Due to the latter, the Royal College of Obstetricians and Gynaecologists Guidelines (RCOG) recommends, based on the National Institute for Health and Care Excellence (NICE) guidelines (2004), IUI treatment without ovarian stimulation, even though it is associated with higher pregnancy rates (Level 1a).

Remarkable is one Level 2 study that demonstrated a significantly higher pregnancy rate and live birth rate in natural cycle IUI for women above 37 years compared to IUI with OH.[5] This difference became even more significant when IUI was combined with stimulation by clomiphene citrate.

Apparently, older women benefit more from natural cycle IUI. This phenomenon might be explained by the age-related decline in ovarian reserve, where the selected dominant follicle represents the best in the cohort, hence increasing the likelihood of fertilization and implantation. Ovarian stimulation could provoke the recruitment of only suboptimal additional follicles that would not have developed in a natural cycle.

We can conclude that female age is an important predictor of pregnancy outcome for couples with unexplained infertility. These results suggest that IUI should be the treatment of choice for couples with unexplained infertility using husband's sperm until a female age of maximally 40 years. For women over 40 years the predicted probabilities of an ongoing pregnancy after IUI are clearly less favorable.

IUI and the Added Value of Ovarian Reserve Testing

Next to female age, ovarian reserve tests (ORT) could be considered as a potential added value in the prediction of IUI treatment outcome. This hypothesis is based on the knowledge that the ovarian aging process varies greatly among women, a variation that will not be unraveled by age alone. However, in infertile couples, the variability may be much more limited as couples may have selected themselves from the highly fertile ones for age, simply by not having achieved a pregnancy in spite of an absent explanation.

Early follicular FSH and antimüllerian hormone (AMH) concentrations are known markers of ovarian reserve and are used in ovarian response prediction to gonadotrophins for *in vitro* fertilization treatment. Much like for the ultrasound assessment of the antral follicle count (AFC), basal FSH and AMH levels are strongly correlated with chronological female age. These three tests, describing mainly quantity aspects of the ovarian aging process, have been mainly studied for their added value in predicting success after IUI treatment.

Current literature offers a limited number of nine papers concerning the predictive value of the ovarian reserve test in IUI treatment. Most studies did not take female age into account properly when analyzing the predictive value of the ORT under study.

TABLE 6.1

Statements of Chapter 6

Statement	Level of Evidence (LOE)
Female age is the only relevant predictor of the probability of pregnancy in IUI treatment	1b
A sharp decline of IUI success rate is observed in women over the age of 40 years, presumably related to oocyte quality	1b
The benefit of OH in IUI treatment remains unclear in older women	1b

TABLE 6.2

Recommendations of Chapter 6

Recommendation	Grade Strength
In couples with unexplained infertility, IUI treatment should be limited to couples with female age under 40 years	A
No routine ovarian reserve screening prior to starting IUI treatment should be advised	B
When using donor semen, IUI may be encouraged to continue up to 42 years	A

In addition to one Level 1b study,[6] the few papers that did evaluate the added value of ORT on top of female age were retrospective cohort studies. Multi-variate analyses for the probability of pregnancy were only performed in four studies, which demonstrated contradictory results for the routine use of ORT prior to IUI treatment. One study showed no significant value for AMH (Level 1b), and the other did not show a significant value for AFC on top of female age in the prediction of pregnancy (Level 3). A third study found a lower AFC to be associated with lower clinical pregnancy rates (Level 3) while the last study described that FSH interacts with age to constitute a useful predictor of pregnancy in women above 34 years (Level 3).

It must therefore be concluded that for application prior to initiating IUI treatment, ovarian reserve tests are of poor predictive value for nonpregnancy in addition to chronological age. This underlines the importance of female age as a strong and useful predictor for successful outcome in IUI treatment.

Current data may suggest that ovarian reserve tests may only be useful to exclude older women from treatment if levels are significantly abnormal and the only effective treatment may be oocyte donation.[1]

The question remains, what gain can be made for a couple to undergo IUI treatment for mild male or unexplained subfertility when the female partner is in her late 30s? Should stimulated IUI treatment be applied in this group, while multi-follicular growth is not desirable and now considered as a complication of the IUI treatment? There may be an argument for counseling these couples directly toward IVF treatment. *In vitro* fertilization (IVF) as an alternative treatment, however, is accompanied by a significant increase in investments of time and money. There are also arguments that ICSI is more effective in unexplained infertility to minimize the risk of total fertilization failure with low numbers of oocytes retrieved, but these results were based on women less than 40 years of age.

REFERENCES

1. Broekmans F.J., Soules M.R., and Fauser B.C. 2009. Ovarian aging: Mechanisms and clinical consequences. *Endocr Rev* August 30(5):465–93.
2. Adamson G.D. and Baker V.L. 2003. Subfertility: Causes, treatment and outcome. *Best Pract Res Clin Obstet Gynaecol* April 17(2):169–85.
3. Verhulst S.M., Cohlen B.J., Hughes E., te Velde E., and Heineman M.J. 2006. Intra-uterine insemination for unexplained subfertility. *Cochrane Database Syst Rev* (4):CD001838.
4. de Brucker M. and Tournaye H. 2010. The effect of age on the outcome of intrauterine insemination: A review. *F, V & V in ObGyn* Monograph:42–50.
5. Kalu E., Thum M.Y., and Abdalla H. 2007. Intrauterine insemination in natural cycle may give better results in older women. *J Assist Reprod Genet* February 24(2–3):83–6.

6. Freiesleben N., Rosendahl M., Johannsen T.H., Lossl K., Loft A., Bangsboll S., et al. 2010. Prospective investigation of serum anti-Mullerian hormone concentration in ovulatory intrauterine insemination patients: A preliminary study. *Reprod Biomed Online* May 20(5):582–7.
7. Harlow S.D., Gass M., Hall J.E., Lobo R., Maki P., Rebar R.W., et al. 2012. Executive summary of the Stages of Reproductive Aging Workshop. *J Clin Endocrinol Metab* April 97(4):1159–68.
8. Hansen K.R., Knowlton N.S., Thyer A.C., Charleston J.S., Soules M.R., and Klein N.A. 2008. A new model of reproductive aging: The decline in ovarian non-growing follicle number from birth to menopause. *Hum Reprod* March 23(3):699–708.
9. de Bruin J.P., Bovenhuis H., van Noord P.A., Pearson P.L., van Arendonk J.A., te Velde E.R., et al. 2001. The role of genetic factors in age at natural menopause. *Hum Reprod* September 16(9):2014–8.

7

Factors Influencing IUI Outcome: Male Age

Michael de Brucker and Herman Tournaye

Delayed Fatherhood[1]

More and more men of older age now father children with their younger partners and the number of men over the age of 35 desiring to conceive children has increased over the past 40 years (Table 7.1: LOE 1b).[1] According to the Office for National Statistics, the mean age of a father at birth in 1971 was 27.2 years but by 1999 this had risen to 30.1 years, and by 2004 it had risen to 32 years. In 2004 in the United Kingdom, more than 75,000 babies, that is, more than one in ten of all newborns, were born to fathers aged 40 years or over, and 6,489 children were born to fathers aged 50 years or over. In the United States in the 1970s, fewer than 15% of all men fathering children were over the age of 35. Today, this percentage has risen to almost 25%. Likewise, there has been a notable increase in the number of men fathering children in their fifties. The discrepancy in the reproductive span between males and females is astonishing and higher reproductive risks associated with advancing maternal age prompt the question whether advanced paternal age too is associated with compromised fertility and increasing risks.

Histology and Sperm Quality[2,3]

Declining reproductive function with aging at the level of the testis has been proven in rodent models. Rats and mice are good animal models for investigating the mechanisms of reproductive aging in males. Aging of rodents appears to be related to histologic changes. Significant changes have been shown and included a decrease in the number of germ cells, a thinning of the seminiferous tubule epithelium, the presence of testicular atrophy, a decrease in sperm motility, and a significantly reduced total sperm production (LOE 1b).[5,6,7] At the histologic level these findings are similar in humans (LOE 2b).[8]

Assessment of semen analyses has been one of the benchmarks for the evaluation of the effect of aging on fertility. Spermatids and spermatocytes disappeared in very old mice (33 months old), and spermatogenesis was severely interrupted. Older mice have atrophied testes, fewer motile sperm, and fail to mate when paired with young females. Significantly reduced total sperm production among older rats (22 and 30 months old) was reported (LOE 1b).[7]

In humans, effects of aging demonstrated a reduction in testicular volume only in the 8th decade of life (LOE 2b).[9] A recent study (LOE 1b)[10] analyzed the effect of male age on sperm analysis by motile sperm organelle morphology examination (MSOME). A consistent decline in semen quality with increasing age was observed. Considering the relationship between nuclear vacuoles and DNA damage, these age-related changes predict that increased paternal age should be associated with unsuccessful or abnormal pregnancy as a consequence. Mechanisms of cell senescence have been well studied in the last decade, and the free radical theory, conceived by Denham Harman in 1956, has attracted considerable attention. The effect of mitochondrial generation of reactive oxygen species (ROS) and aging on human spermatozoa and seminal antioxidants was discussed in a review in 2010 (LOE 1b).[11] ROS are continually produced in the mitochondria and play an important role in age-related male pathophysiology. The increased

ROS level in semen observed with aging is associated with a possible decrease in antioxidant enzyme activity. This imbalance between pro-oxidants and antioxidants induces oxidative damage, resulting in abnormalities in telomeres and telomerase in male germline cells. This sequence of events may explain the decrease in sperm concentration seen with aging. Oxidative stress may inhibit sperm axonemal phosphorylation and increase lipid peroxidation, which can decrease sperm motility. This oxidative stress can also lead to lipofuscin and amyloid accumulation in the male reproductive tract, potentially the cause of decreased Leydig cell function and a subsequent decrease in blood testosterone levels. Along with its negative effect on the fertilizing potential of spermatozoa, ROS also leads to offspring malformation. Oxidative stress-induced mtDNA damage and nuclear DNA damage in aging men may put them at a higher risk for transmitting multiple genetic and chromosomal defects (see Table 7.2).

A review over a 20 year period compared the semen quality of 50-year-old men with 30-year-old men (LOE 2a).[12] There was a 3–22% decrease in semen volume, a 3–37% decrease in sperm motility, and a 4–18% decrease in normal sperm concentration. The weight of the evidence suggests that increased male age is associated with a decline in semen volume, sperm motility, and sperm morphology but *not* with sperm concentration. Among studies that did control for female age, relative decreases in pregnancy rates were found in men over 50. Changes observed in semen quality can be associated by two mechanisms. First, there may be cellular and/or physiological changes in the genitourinary tract with aging. In autopsies of men who died from accidental causes, there have been seen age-related narrowing and sclerosis of the testicular tubular lumen, decreases in spermatogenetic activity, increased degeneration of germ cells, and decreased numbers and function of Leydig cells (LOE 2b).[13,14] Decreased semen volume with age may be caused by seminal vesicle insufficiency, since seminal vesicle fluid contributes most of the ejaculate volume.[15,16] Changes in the prostate that occur with aging, such as smooth muscle atrophy and a decrease in protein and water content, may contribute to decreased semen volume and sperm motility. In addition, there may be age-related changes in the epididymis where sperm acquire the capacity for vigorous forward motility during transit. The epididymis is a hormonally sensitive tissue, which plays an important role in sperm maturation. Thus, hormonal or epididymal senescence may lead to decreased motility in older men. Second, aging is associated with reproductive damage due to an increase in male accessory gland infections in men.[1]

Increasing Age, Declining Fertility?[3,4]

Semen parameters start to decline after 35 years of age. Male fertility was found to decrease substantially in the late 30s and continues to decrease after age 40 while controlling for female age (LOE 1b).[17] Nevertheless, in contrast to female fertility, male fertility is maintained until very late in life, and, in addition to anecdotal reports, it has been documented up to an age of 94 years (LOE 4).[18] Age-dependent decrease of fertility in couples is usually attributed to female aging, which makes studies on a male age effect difficult. In addition to female age, further confounders, such as reduced coital frequency, an increasing incidence of erectile dysfunction, and smoking habits have to be considered. For natural conception, paternal age has a limited effect whenever the female partner is young. Time to pregnancy is longer than compared to younger men. However, when the female partner too is of age, then a synergistic adverse effect of paternal age is observed (LOE 2b).[4]

Impact of Male Aging on IUI Success Rates

With methods of assisted reproduction, factors interfering with natural conception, for example, concentration or motility, may be circumvented. The more invasive the treatment, the less important male age appears: success rates of IVF or ICSI are not affected by male age. On the other hand, the success rate of intra-uterine insemination (IUI) is affected by male age, probably because IUI requires sperm of much higher quality than for IVF/ICSI (LOE 2b).[19,20]

Yet, data on male aging and IUI success rates are limited. After controlling for maternal age, paternal age over 35 years is an important predictive factor of success. A 50% lower pregnancy rate was observed

TABLE 7.1

Statements of Chapter 7

Statement	Level of Evidence (LOE)
Increased male age seems to be associated with a decline in semen volume, sperm motility and sperm morphology but *not* with sperm concentration	2a
Semen parameters start to decline after 35 years of age	1b*
Paternal age seems to have no profound effect when the female partner is younger than 35 years	2b
A synergistic adverse effect seems to exist when the female partner is older than 35 years beyond a male age over 35 years	2a
Oxidative stress-induced mtDNA damage and nuclear DNA damage in aging men may put them at a higher risk for transmitting multiple genetic and chromosomal defects	2b

* From Kühnert B. and Nieschlag E., 2004, *Hum Reprod Update* 10(4):327–39; Stewart A.F. and Kim E.D., 2011, *Urology* 78(3):496–9; Tournaye H., 2009, In: *Reproductive Aging,* London: RCOG Press, 89–94; De La Rochebrochard E., McElreavey K., and Thonneau P., 2003, *J Androl* 24(4):459–65.

TABLE 7.2

Recommendations of Chapter 7

Recommendation	Grade Strength
Men with a female partner above 35 years should be informed that increasing paternal age (40 years and above) has a potential negative impact on IUI success rates	A

when the male partner was older than 35 years in comparison to males 30 years or younger. It seems that paternal age only has an influence in case of maternal age of 35 years and above (LOE 2b).[19] This age cut-off is not so surprising since maternal age over 35 years is a well-known risk factor for miscarriages. In contrast, one large retrospective trial concluded that this paternal age effect was observed in all female age groups (LOE 2b).[21] Although more than 17,000 IUI cycles were analyzed, this study did not properly control for confounding factors including maternal age and hence the conclusions remain debatable. We may suggest that paternal age has no impact on IUI success rates as long as the female partner is less than 35 years. Furthermore, paternal age above 40 years seems to be a risk factor as well for spontaneous abortion (LOE 2b).[22]

Impact of male aging in IUI combined with human menopausal gonadotrophin (hMG) has been studied as well. The clinical pregnancy rate was significantly lower in males aged 40 years or older compared with males aged less than 40 years when their female partners were 35 years or older (16.3% versus 6.5%, P = 0.02). However, no differences were observed when female partners were less than 35 years. Also, this study concluded that a synergistic adverse effect seems to exist when the female partner is older than 35 years beyond a male age over 35 years (LOE 2b).[23]

REFERENCES

1. Kühnert B. and Nieschlag E. 2004. Reproductive functions of the aging male. *Hum Reprod Update* July–August 10(4):327–339 [Epub: 2004, June 10, Review].
2. Stewart A.F. and Kim E.D. 2011. Fertility concerns for the aging male. *Urology* September 78(3):496–499, Review.
3. Tournaye H. 2009. Male reproductive aging. In: *Reproductive Aging,* eds. Bewley S., Ledger W., Nikolaou D. London: RCOG Press, 89–94, Review.
4. De La Rochebrochard E., McElreavey K., and Thonneau P. 2003. Paternal age over 40 years: The "amber light" in the reproductive life of men? *J Androl* July–August 24(4):459–465, Review.
5. Tanemura K., Kurohmaru M., Kuramoto K., and Hayashi Y. 1993. Age-related morphological changes in the testis of the BDF1 mouse. *J Vet Med Sci* October 55(5):703–710.

6. Parkening T.A., Collins T.J., and Au W.W. 1988. Paternal age and its effects on reproduction in C57BL/6NNia mice. *J Gerontol* May 43(3):B79–B84.

7. Wang C., Hikim A.S., Ferrini M., Bonavera J.J., Vernet D., Leung A., Lue Y.H., Gonzalez-Cadavid N.F., and Swerdloff R.S. 1993. Male reproductive ageing: Using the brown Norway rat as a model for man. *Endocrinology* 133(6):2773–2781.

8. Dakouane M., Bicchieray L., Bergere M., Albert M., Vialard F., and Selva J. 2005. A histomorphometric and cytogenetic study of testis from men 29–102 years old. *Fertil Steril* April 83(4):923–928.

9. Handelsman D.J. and Starj S. 1985. Testicular size: The effects of aging, malnutrition, and illness. *J Androl* 6(6):144–151.

10. Silva L.F., Oliveira J.B., Petersen C.G., Mauri A.L., Massaro F.C., Cavagna M., Baruffi R.L., and Franco J.G. Jr. 2012. The effects of male age on sperm analysis by motile sperm organelle morphology examination (MSOME). *Reprod Biol Endocrinol* March 10(1):19 [Epub ahead of print].

11. Desai N., Sabanegh E. Jr., Kim T., and Agarwal A. 2010. Free radical theory of aging: Implications in male infertility. 2010. *Urology* January 75(1):14–19. doi: 10.1016/j.urology.2009.05.025 [Epub July 17, 2009, Review].

12. Kidd S.A., Eskenazi B., and Wyrobek A.J. 2001. Effects of male age on semen quality and fertility: A review of the literature. *Fertil Steril* February 75(2):237–248, Review.

13. Bishop M.W. 1970. Ageing and reproduction in the male. *J Reprod Fertil* (Suppl.) March 12:65–87.

14. Johnson L. Spermatogenesis and aging in the human. 1986. *J Androl* November–December 7(6):331–354.

15. Hamilton D. and Naftolin F. 1981. *Basis Reproductive Medicine*. Cambridge, UK: MIT Press.

16. Goldman N. and Montgomery M. 1989. Fecundability and husband's age. *Soc Biol* (36):146–166.

17. Dunson D.B., Baird D.D., and Colombo B. 2004. Increased infertility with age in men and women. *Obstet Gynecol* January 103(1):51–56.

18. Seymour F.I. 1935. A case of authenticated fertility in a man aged 94. *JAMA*105:1423–1424.

19. Mathieu C., Ecochard R., Bied V., Lornage J., and Czyba J.C. 1995. Cumulative conception rate following intrauterine artificial insemination with husband's spermatozoa: Influence of husband's age. *Hum Reprod* May 10(5):1090–7.

20. Brzechffa P.R. and Buyalos R.P. 1997. Female and male partner age and menotrophin requirements influence pregnancy rates with human menopausal gonadotropin therapy in combination with intrauterine insemination. *Hum Reprod* January 12(1):29–33.

21. Belloc S., Cohen-Bacrie P., Benkhalifa M., Cohen-Bacrie M., De Mouzon J., Hazout A., and Ménézo Y. 2008. Effect of maternal and paternal age on pregnancy and miscarriage rates after intrauterine insemination. *Reprod Biomed Online* September 17(3):392–397.

22. De La Rochebrochard E. and Thonneau P. 2002. Paternal age and maternal age are risk factors for miscarriage: Results of a multi-centre European study. *Hum Reprod* June 17(6):1649–1656.

23. Brzechffa P.R. and Buyalos R.P. 1997. Female and male partner age and menotrophin requirements influence pregnancy rates with human menopausal gonadotrophin therapy in combination with intrauterine insemination. *Hum Reprod* January 12(1):29–33.

8

Factors Influencing IUI Outcome: Weight Influences

John C. Petrozza, Irene Dimitriadis, and Pratap Kumar

Intra-uterine insemination (IUI) is a procedure performed to facilitate fertilization. It involves placing sperm inside a woman's uterus without manipulating her eggs and therefore is not categorized as an assisted reproductive technology (ART) procedure. The decision to use this fertility treatment depends on the couple's infertility diagnosis and works best in women whose cervix prevents sperm from entering the uterine cavity and in men when the majority of their sperm is immotile. IUI success rates can be as high as 20% per cycle depending on a variety of factors such as the use of fertility medications, age of the female partner, and infertility diagnosis, as well as other factors that may impact the success of the cycle.[1]

Total body fat has been linked to the risk of disease and death. Body mass index (BMI) has proven to be a good indicator of total body fat, although it tends to overestimate body fat in individuals who have a muscular build (e.g., athletes) and underestimate it in those who have lost muscle mass (e.g., elderly). Weighing too much or too little has been shown to interrupt the normal menstrual cycle. Extreme BMIs, either high or low, can throw off ovulation or even stop it all together. Abdominal adiposity (fat around the waist and chest, also known as apple shape), and in particular belly fat, has been linked to ovulatory problems via inflammatory molecules that are secreted in the gut.[2–4]

There is a developing, yet controversial, amount of evidence suggesting that obesity is associated with lower oocyte yield with gonadotrophin stimulation, lower clinical pregnancy rates, and an increase in pregnancy loss in patients undergoing *in vitro* fertilization treatment.[5–12] Even less certain is the effect of obesity on ovulation induction and insemination.

The disparity in these results can be attributed to many factors that were not often controlled in these studies. These include types of treatment, patient heterogeneity, inconsistent definitions of obesity, influence of spousal obesity on pregnancy rates, and the increased prevalence of obesity on ovulatory rates. In addition, primary and secondary end points are often different among the studies, making comparisons very difficult. More importantly, these *in vitro* fertilization studies often neglected comparisons to infertile control groups, specifically those patients undergoing simple ovulation induction cycles.

One of the first reports describing the effect of weight on ovulation induction and pregnancy rates was in 2004, when Wang and colleagues reported pregnancy rates that increased from 19.2% in underweight patients to 38% in obese patients.[13] Patients' infertility criteria were not well defined, and it was suggested that many of the obese women were simply anovulatory and thus were able to conceive easily once they ovulated with gonadotrophin therapy.

Dodson and colleagues in 2006 reviewed 333 women in a retrospective chart review who had undergone ovulation induction and IUI for infertility.[14] The women had normal menstrual cycles based on history and elevated luteal progesterone levels, at least one patent fallopian tube, and total motile sperm concentration for each IUI was at least 1 million. Follicle-stimulating hormone was used for ovarian stimulation using 150–225 units and cycles were canceled if the estradiol went above 2000 pg/ml, progesterone levels suggested premature luteinization, or greater than seven pre-ovulatory follicles developed. These are clearly liberal guidelines by many standards and perhaps represent patient records that were reviewed from the early 1990s, which also suggest different gonadotrophin preparations and protocols over the 14 years (1990–2004) charts were reviewed for this study. However, adjusting for year did not alter results.

The mean patient age was 33.2 +/– 4.4 years and patient diagnoses ranged from idiopathic to male factor. Women were divided into four body mass index (BMI, kg/m^2) categories: <18.5 (underweight), 18.5 to <25 (normal), 25 to <30 (overweight), >=30 (obese). The larger the BMI, the more gonadotrophins the patient needed to achieve the same follicular response (approximately 3.5 follicles) yet obese women failed to obtain the same estradiol level as patients with lower BMIs. Despite this, there was no difference in fecundity between all BMI groups (approximately 15%). (See Tables 8.1 and 8.2.)

In a subsequent study in 2011, Souter and colleagues[15] reviewed all patients that had undergone gonadotrophin-IUI cycles over a three-year period (2004–2007), representing more contemporary stimulation protocols and consistent medication types. A total of 1,189 cycles were reviewed from 477 women. Similar BMI categories as in prior studies were analyzed. Obese patients required more gonadotrophins and achieved lower peak estradiol levels, confirming prior studies, and also had similar preovulatory follicles (>15 mm). Compared to the study by Dodson, estradiol and follicular numbers were all relatively lower, reflecting a more conservative approach. Nevertheless, fecundity rates were actually higher in the obese (35.9%) and overweight (37.4%) categories compared to the normal group (24.7%). These numbers did not change even when excluding patients with polycystic ovarian syndrome from the analysis. Endometrial thickness remained stable between patients in all three weight categories. In addition, miscarriage rates between the groups were not significantly different (12%). Interestingly, obese patients were able to conceive in the same number of cycles (1.8) compared to normal weight patients with a statistical trend toward a shorter duration.

Letrozole is an aromatase inhibitor and has emerged in the recent literature as an alternative to clomiphene citrate (CC) for ovulation induction due to its fewer side effects and lower reported rates of multiples. McKnight et al.[16] studied the pregnancy rates among normal weight and obese infertile women undergoing ovulation induction (OI) with letrozole and found a trend for better outcomes in women with a higher BMI.

Thus, compared to the debate in patients undergoing *in vitro* fertilization, elevated BMI does not appear to be associated with a negative effect on treatment outcomes. It is important to realize that these three studies on ovulation induction are all retrospective. Other studies have shown that obesity is associated with increased gonadotrophin requirements, reduced follicular development, and lower oocyte yield. It is unclear why obese patients require higher doses of gonadotrophins, however, it may be related to decreased absorption, altered distribution, and diminished metabolic clearance due to excess fat.[17,18] Additionally, leptin, a cofactor in many regulatory processes, is elevated in the follicular fluid and serum in obese women.[19] Leptin has been shown to suppress granulosa cell production of estradiol by inhibiting ovarian steroidogenesis.[20–22]

Souter et al.[15] also noted a positive association between BMI and endometrial thickness. The latter was positively associated with pregnancy. Trends toward thicker endometrial lines in women with a higher BMI have been reported in other studies as well. This can lead to the hypothesis that any adverse effects of excess weight on the endometrium may be a result of metabolic and hormonal disturbances, embryo uterine dialogue, and altered receptivity rather than linking them to the thickness of the endometrium.[23–25]

Despite the findings that support comparable success rates of obese women treated with gonadotrophins and IUI to those of normal weight women, physicians are encouraged to counsel their patients to optimize their weight before initiating fertility treatment plans. It has been suggested that the best range for natural fertility is a BMI of 20 to 24.[3] Many fertility practices have a minimum and a maximum BMI, in order for a patient to qualify for OI/IUI treatment, not as much to influence pregnancy rates, but primarily to reduce the known obstetrical risks associated with extreme weight.[26,27] With this in mind, it is not clear whether weight loss prior to treatment has a detrimental effect on outcomes. Indeed, a report in 2006 by Tsagareli and colleagues[28] in Australia suggest that a low calorie diet in overweight or obese patients for a short period of time prior to IVF treatment worsened outcomes.

In summary, the influence of weight on IUI outcomes is not yet clear. BMI has proven to be a "practical indicator" of obesity. However, other measures of obesity such as abdominal circumference, waist-to-hip ratio, body fat mass, or trunk–leg fat ratio may need to be considered as potentially more predictive

TABLE 8.1

Statements of Chapter 8

Statement	Level of Evidence (LOE)
Obesity is associated with lower oocyte yield with gonadotrophin stimulation, lower clinical pregnancy rates, and increased pregnancy loss in patients undergoing IVF	2b
In women undergoing gonadotrophin-IUI treatment, fecundity rates are higher in obese patients, even when controlling for women with Polycystic Ovarian Syndrome (PCOS)	3
In women undergoing gonadotrophin-IUI treatment, miscarriage rates are not significantly higher in patients who are obese, compared to women with normal BMIs	3
Decreasing BMI prior to starting a gonadotrophin cycle has not been shown to improve fecundity rates	3

TABLE 8.2

Recommendations of Chapter 8

Recommendation	Grade Strength
In women undergoing gonadotrophin-IUI treatment, the same BMI guidelines used for IVF cannot be applied	C
Recommending weight loss may not improve fecundity, but will improve obstetrical outcomes	B
The optimal BMI for natural fecundity may be between 20–24	D

of the effects of weight on the response to fertility treatment.[3] In addition, these studies suggest that an underweight BMI may also be associated with poor fertility and obstetrical outcomes. Advice to patients should be focused not only on ensuring optimal treatment outcomes, but also promoting the best obstetrical outcomes and ensuring appropriate reinforcement for a healthy lifestyle.

REFERENCES

1. Intrauterine Insemination. 2012. American Society of Reproductive Medicine. http://www.asrm .org/uploadedFiles/ASRM_Content/Resources/Patient_Resources/Fact_Sheets_and_Info_Booklets/ IUI_3-19-12_FINAL.pdf, Revised 2012.
2. World Health Organization (WHO). 2000. Obesity: Preventing and managing the global epidemic: Report of a WHO consultation. Geneva, Switzerland: World Health Organization (Technical report series no. 894).
3. Chavarro J.E., Willett W.C., and Skerrett P.J. 2008. *The Fertility Diet: Groundbreaking Research Reveals Natural Ways to Boost Ovulation & Improve Your Chances of Getting Pregnant.* Boston: McGraw-Hill. 153–216.
4. Wang Y. and Beydoun M.A. 2007. The obesity epidemic in the United States—Gender, age, socioeconomic, racial/ethnic, and geographic characteristics: A systematic review and meta-regression analysis. *Epidemiologic Reviews* 29:6–28.
5. Fedorcsák P., Dale P.O., Storeng R., Ertzeid G., Bjercke S., Oldereid N., Omland A.K., Abyholm T., and Tanbo T. 2004. Impact of overweight and underweight on assisted reproduction treatment. *Hum Reprod.* November 19(11):2523–8.
6. Uhlíková P., Papezová H., Malá E., Valenotvá D., and Rezábek K. 2006. Assisted reproduction in patients with food intake disorders—Clinical and ethical aspects. *Ceska Gynekol.* July 71(4):339–41.
7. Metwally M., Ong K.J., Ledger W.L., and Li T.C. 2008. Does high body mass index increase the risk of miscarriage after spontaneous and assisted conception? A meta-analysis of the evidence. *Fertil Steril* 90:714–26.
8. Dechaud H., Anahory T., Reyftmann L., Loup V., Hamamah S., and Hedon B. 2006. Obesity does not adversely affect results in patients undergoing *in vitro* fertilization and embryo transfer. *Eur J Obstet Gynecol Reprod Biol* 127:88–93.

9. Maheshwari A., Stofberg L., and Bhattacharya S. 2007. Effect of overweight and obesity on assisted reproductive technology—A systematic review. *Hum Reprod Update* 13:433–44.

10. Spandorfer S.D., Kump L., Goldschlag D., Brodkin T., Davis O.K., and Rosenwaks Z. 2004. Obesity and *in vitro* fertilization: Negative influences on outcome. *J Reprod Med* 49:973–7.

11. Matalliotakis I., Cakmak H., Sakkas D., Mahutte N., Koumantakis G., and Arici A. 2008. Impact of body mass index on IVF and ICSI outcome: A retrospective study. *Reprod Biomed Online* 16:778–83.

12. Wattanakumtornkul S., Demario M.A., Stevens Hall S.A., Thornhill A.R., and Tummon I.S. 2003. Body mass index and uterine receptivity in the oocyte donation model. *Fertil Steril* 80:336–40.

13. Wang J.X., Warnes G.W., Davies M.J., and Norman R.J. 2004. Overweight infertile patients have a higher fecundity than normal-weight women undergoing controlled ovarian hyperstimulation with intra-uterine insemination. *Fertil Steril* June 81(6):1710–12.

14. Dodson W.C., Kunselman A.R., and Legro R.S. 2006. Association of obesity with treatment outcomes in ovulatory infertile women undergoing superovulation and intrauterine insemination. *Fertil Steril* September 86(3):642–6.

15. Souter I., Baltagi L.M., Kuleta D., Meeker J.D., and Petrozza J.C. 2011. Women, weight, and fertility: The effect of body mass index on the outcome of superovulation/intrauterine insemination cycles. *Fertil Steril* March 195(3):1042–7.

16. McKnight K.K., Nodler J.L., Cooper J.J. Jr., Chapman V.R., Cliver S.P., and Bates G.W. Jr. 2011. Body mass index-associated differences in response to ovulation induction with letrozole. *Fertil Steril* November 96(5):1206–8.

17. Steinkampf M.P., Moilanen J.M., Lehtovirta M., Tuomi T., Hovatta O., Siegberg R. et al. 2003. Effect of obesity on recombinant follicle-stimulating hormone absorption: Subcutaneous versus intramuscular administration. *Fertil Steril* 80:99–101.

18. Balen A.H., Plattau P., Andersen A.N., Devroey P., Sorensen P., Halmgaard L. et al. 2006. The influence of body weight on response to ovulation induction with gonadotrophins in 335 women with World Health Organization group II anovulatory infertility. *Br J Obstet Gynecol* 113:1195–202.

19. Castellucci M., De Matteis R., Meisser A., Cancello R., Monsurro V., Islami D. et al. 2000. Leptin modulates extracellular matrix molecules and metalloproteinases: Possible implications for trophoblast invasion. *Mol Hum Reprod* 6:951–8.

20. Gonzalez R.R., Caballero-Campo P., Jaspar M., Mercader A., Devoto L., Pllicer A. et al. 2000. Leptin and leptin receptor are expressed in the human endometrium and endometrial leptin secretion is regulated by the human blastocyst. *J Clin Endocrinol Metab* 85:4883–8.

21. Agarwal S.K., Vogel K., Weitsman S.R., and Magoffin D.A. 1999. Leptin antagonizes the insulin-like growth factor-I augmentation of steroidogenesis in granulosa and theca cells of the human ovary. *J Clin Endocrinol Metab* 84:1072–6.

22. Ghizzoni L., Barreca A., Mastorakos G., Furlini M., Vottero A., Ferrari B. et al. 2001. Leptin inhibits steroid biosynthesis by human granulosa-lutein cells. *Horm Metab Res* 33:323–8.

23. Bellver J., Melo M.A., Bosch E., Serra V., Remohi J., and Pellicier A. 2007. Obesity and poor reproductive outcome: The potential role of the endometrium. *Fertil Steril* 88:446–51.

24. Erel C.T. and Senturk L.M. 2009. The impact of body mass index on assisted reproduction. *Curr Opin Obstet Gynecol* 21:228–35.

25. Metwally M., Tuckerman E.M., Laird S.M., Ledger W.L., and Li T.C. 2007. Impact of high body mass index on endometrial morphology and function in the peri-implantation period in women with recurrent miscarriage. *Reprod Biomed Online* 14:328–34.

26. Yu C.K., Teoh T.G., and Robinson S. 2006. Obesity in pregnancy. *Br J Obstet Gynecol* 333:1117–25.

27. Dietl J. 2005. Maternal obesity and complications during pregnancy. *J Perinatl Med* 33:100–5.

28. Tsagareli V., Noakes M., and Norman R.J. 2006. Effect of a very low-calorie-diet on *in vitro* fertilization outcomes. *Fertil Steril.* July 86(1):227–9.

9

Factors Influencing IUI Outcome: Semen Quality

Willem Ombelet, Nathalie Dhont, and Thinus Kruger

Introduction

It is generally accepted that intra-uterine insemination (IUI) should be preferred to more invasive and expensive techniques of assisted reproduction and be offered as a first choice treatment in case of unexplained and/or moderate male factor subfertility.

Scientific validation of this strategy is difficult because the literature is rather confusing and not conclusive. To find out which couples can benefit from IUI in case of male infertility we need to investigate the power of different semen parameters in predicting success after IUI. Although the World Health Organization tried to standardize the performances of semen analysis and related procedures in order to reduce variation in the results obtained, a literature search on this topic is frustrating due to the ongoing lack of standardization in interpretation of semen results.[1]

A literature search was performed to investigate the threshold levels of sperm parameters above which IUI pregnancy outcome is significantly improved or the cut-off values reach substantial discriminative performance in an IUI program.[2]

Methods

Search Strategy

By means of a computerized MEDLINE search we reviewed the literature for a 30 year period, from 1982 to 2011. We used the following keywords: (success or outcome or pregnancy or predictive value) AND (semen or sperm) AND (IUI). Other relevant studies were identified by searching EMBASE and Cochrane Controlled Trial Register published until December 2011. We also looked at the reference lists of the selected articles.

Study Inclusion Criteria and Data Extraction

Studies were only included if they reported on the value of sperm parameters on the prediction of IUI success in couples with male subfertility. Only studies with a minimum of 200 IUI cycles using homologous sperm were included. Male subfertility was defined by semen quality below the standards of the World Health Organization during that specific period. The outcome most frequently used was clinical pregnancy defined as a pregnancy confirmed by a gestational sac and/or fetal heart activity on ultrasound. At present, results are mostly expressed as live birth rates or ongoing pregnancy rates per couple applying intention to treat analysis. Unfortunately these outcome parameters were not used in the selected studies.

Results

In the Cochrane Library, 10 reviews could be selected; in none of these reviews were the predictive value of semen parameters and IUI outcome were evaluated. Our EMBASE and MEDLINE search revealed a total of 983 papers. Only 53 studies (5.4%) fulfilled our inclusion criteria and these papers were analyzed (Table 9.3). A retrospective analysis was performed in 34 papers; in 13 articles the results of a prospective observational study were described. Last but not least we found five structured reviews and/ or meta-analyses. Van Waart et al.[3] and Ombelet et al.[4] concluded that a score of more than 4% normal morphology using strict criteria was needed to result in a significantly higher pregnancy rate per cycle. In the meta-analysis of Van Waart et al.,[3] six studies yielded a risk difference (RD) between the pregnancy rates achieved in the patients below and above the 4% strict criteria threshold of −0.07 (95% CI: −0.11 to 4.03; P<0.001). In the meta-analysis of 16 studies by Van Weert et al.,[5] receiver operating characteristics (ROC) curves indicated a reasonable predictive performance toward IUI outcome for the Inseminating Motile Count (IMC) (Figure 9.1). At cut-off levels between 0.8 to 5 million the specificity of the IMC, defined as the ability to predict failure to become pregnant, was as high as 100%; the sensitivity of the test, defined as the ability to predict pregnancy, was limited.

According to Ombelet et al.,[6] an IMC of 1 million can be used as a reasonable threshold level above which IUI can be performed with acceptable pregnancy rates. Overall, sperm morphology and IMC were of no prognostic value using ROC curve analysis. Sperm morphology turned out to be a valuable prognostic parameter in predicting IUI success if the IMC was less than 1 million (area under ROC curve: 77.6%). The cumulative live birth rate (CLBR) after three IUI cycles was 13.6% if the IMC was less than 1 million, significantly different from the group with an IMC >1 million (22.4%, p<0.05). Considering only patients with IMC <1 million and sperm morphology >4%, the CLBR was 21.9%, comparable with the CLBR of all cycles with an IMC of more than 1 million.[6]

The four sperm parameters that were most frequently examined and cited were the following: (a) the IMC, (b) sperm morphology using strict criteria, (c) the TMSC (total motile sperm count in the native sperm sample), and (d) the TM (total motility in the native sperm sample).

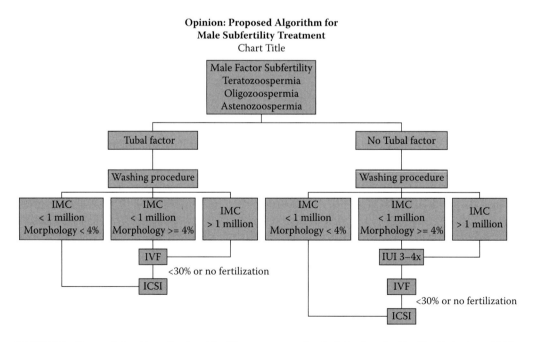

FIGURE 9.1   Proposed algorithm of male subfertility treatment at the Genk Institute for Fertility Technology (IMC = Inseminating Motile Count).

TABLE 9.3

Overview of Papers Examining and Reporting on the Influence of Sperm Quality on IUI Outcome (Period 1982–2011)

Year	First Author	Country	Couples (n)	Cycles (n)	Sperm Parameter	Threshold	Type of Study
2011	Yang	China	482	—	SCSA-DFI	<25%	POS
2011	Demir	Turkey	212	253	TMSC	>10 mill	RA
					Morphology SC	>4%	
2011	Youn	China	—	383	CASA Conc	111 mill	RA
					CASA Mot AB	51.40%	
					CASA Mot A	30.10%	
2011	Dorjpurev	Japan	283	1177	TM	>30%	RA
					TMSC	>10 mill	
2011	Nikbakht	Iran	445	820	TMSC	5–10 mill	POS
					IMC	>10 mill	
					Morphology SC	≥5%	
2010	Merviel	France	138	353	TMSC	>5 mill	RA
2010	Castilla	Spain	—	—	SCSA-DFI	—	Structured review
2010	Tijani	United Kingdom	—	—	TMSC	>10 mill	Structured review
2009	Haim	France	—	248	Mot A	>10%	POS
2009	Badawy	Egypt	393	714	IMC	>5 mill	POS
					Morphology WHO	>30%	
2008	De la Cuesta	Spain	183	500	IMC	>1.5 mill	RA
2008	Guven	Turkey	232	255	Morphology SC	>4%	RA
2007	Bungum	Denmark	—	387	SCSA-DFI	<=30%	RA
2007	Tay	Malaysia	317	507	IMC / TMSC	>20 mill	RA
2007	Kdous	Tunisia	138	206	IMC	>1.1 mill	RA
2006	Mehrannia	Iran	824	824	IMC	>10 mill	RA
2006	Arslan	United States	82	313	HZI	<30%	POS
2005	Grigoriou	Greece	615	1641	Morphology SC	>10%	RA
2004	Van Weert	The Netherlands	—	—	IMC	0.8–5 mill	Meta-analysis
2004	Zhao	United States	431	1007	TM	>80%	RA
2004	Yalti	Turkey	190	268	TM	>30%	RA
2004	Wainer	France	889	2564	IMC + Morphology WHO	>5 mill/ >30%	RA
2004	Shibahara	Japan	160	682	Morphology SC	>15.5%	POS
					CASA-RASP	>=25.5%	
2004	De la Cuesta	Spain	168	430	IMC	>2 mill	RA
2003	Saucedo	Spain	—	787	Morphology WHO	>20%	RA
					IMC	>1 mill	
2003	Ombelet	Belgium	—	—	Morphology SC	>4%	Structured review
					IMC	>1 mill	
2003	Makkar	Hong Kong	292	600	IC	>20 mill/mL	RA
					Morphology SC	≥7%	
					IMC	>1 mill	
2002	Miller	United States	438	1114	IMC	>10 mill	POS

(Continued)

TABLE 9.3 (*Continued*)

Overview of Papers Examining and Reporting on the Influence of Sperm Quality on IUI Outcome (Period 1982–2011)

Year	First Author	Country	Couples (n)	Cycles (n)	Sperm Parameter	Threshold	Type of Study
2002	Lee	Singapore	1479	2846	IMC	>1 mill	RA
					TM	>30%	
2002	Lee	China	209	244	Morphology SC	>4%	POS
2001	Montanaro	South Africa	—	495	Morphology SC	>4%	RA
2001	Van Voorhis	United States	1039	3479	TMSC	>10 mill	RA
					TM	>50%	
2001	Khalil	Denmark	893	2473	IMC	>5 mill	RA
2001	Hauser	Israel	108	264	Morphology SC	>4%	POS
2001	Van Waart	South Africa	—	—	Morphology SC	>4%	Structured review
1999	Dickey	United States	1841	4056	Mot AB	≥30%	RA
					TC	≥10 mill	
					TMSC	≥5 mill	
1999	Stone	United States	—	9963	TMSC	≥4 mill	RA
					TM	≥60%	
1999	Branigan	United States	414	1100	IMC	≥10 mill	POS
					Sperm survival 24 h	≥70%	
1998	Van der Westerlaken	The Netherlands	566	1763	IMC	>10 mill	RA
1998	Shulman	Israel	160	544	Semen parameters	Not useful	RA
1997	Ombelet	Belgium	373	792	IMC & Morphology SC	>1 mill + >4%	RA
1997	Karabinus	United States	193	538	Morphology SC	Not useful	RA
1997	Berg	Germany	902	3037	IMC	>0.8 mill	RA
1996	Ombelet	Belgium	412	1100	Morphology SC	≥4%	RA
1996	Huang	China	939	1375	IMC	>5 mill	POS
1996	Campana	Switzerland	332	1115	IMC	>1 mill	POS
1996	Burr	Australia	163	330	Morphology SC	>10%	RA
					IMC	Not useful	
1995	Toner	United States	126	395	IMC	>2 mill	RA
					Morphology SC	>4%	
1995	Matorras	Spain	74	271	Morphology SC	Not useful	POS
1994	Brasch	United States	546	1205	IMC	>20 mill	RA
1990	Francavilla	Italy	86	411	Morphology WHO	>50%	RA
					TMSC	>5 mill	
1989	Horvath	United States	232	451	IMC	>1 mill	RA

Note: POS = prospective observational study, RA = retrospective analysis, IMC = Inseminating Motile Count or postwash total motile sperm count, Morphology SC = morphology according to strict criteria, Morphology WHO = morphology according to WHO criteria, TMSC = Total Motile Sperm Count native sperm sample, TM = Total Motility native sperm sample, Mot AB = grade a + b motility, Mot A = grade a motility, IC = Initial Concentration native sperm sample, SCSA-DFI = Sperm Chromatin Structure Assay-DNA Fragmentation Index, CASA = Computer Assisted Sperm Analysis, HZI = Hemizona Index.

In 20 articles, the IMC was cited as an important predictive parameter, in 8 out of 20 studies a cut-off value of 1 million was mentioned, in four studies between 1 and 2 million, in five studies the authors calculated a threshold value of 5 million.

Sperm morphology using strict criteria was the second most cited sperm parameter. In 11 out of 15 studies, 4% normal forms was reported as the best cut-off value. When utilizing these cut-off values of sperm morphology and IMC, there is poor sensitivity for predicting who will conceive but a high specificity for predicting failure to conceive with IUI.

The TMSC was also reported to be an important predictive parameter in 10 papers with a cut-off value of 5 million in five papers and 10 million in four papers. A TM threshold value of 30% was found in three out of six articles in which the TM was found to be a good predictor of success.

Discussion

Until today no prospective cohort trial investigating the predicting value of semen parameters on IUI outcome by using ROC curves and multi-variate analyses has been published. As a result of our literature search we have to admit that our calculations are based on Level 2 to Level 3 evidence. Nevertheless, it seems that the following cut-off values can be used when talking about semen parameters with an important and substantial discriminative performance in an IUI program: IMC >1 million, sperm morphology using strict criteria >4%, a TMSC of more than 5 million, and a TM of more than 30%. It does not mean that below these cut-off levels IUI cannot be used as a good and effective first-line treatment in male subfertility cases, it only tells us that above these threshold levels the success rate after IUI seems to be significantly better.

It is obvious that many other factors may influence the impact of sperm quality on IUI success. Among these factors the duration of subfertility, the female age, and the use of ovarian stimulation protocols are well recognized to be associated with IUI success, indirectly influencing the impact of semen quality on IUI outcome.

The lack of large prospective cohort studies is easy to understand. Because natural cycle IUI and clomiphene citrate stimulation are frequently used in an IUI program, the budget of IUI treatment is almost neglectable when compared to the budget spent on other methods of assisted reproduction such as IVF and ICSI. Studies supported and organized by the pharmaceutical industry are not available and in most cases even the governments are not interested at all.

We believe that well-organized randomized studies are urgently needed to define usable cut-off values for selecting couples for IUI in male subfertility cases, taking into account cost-effectiveness of the different methods of assisted reproduction.[7]

If we look into the future, we can expect a marked increase in pregnancy rates with IVF compared to IUI, in general. Recent studies modeling outcomes and costs showed that moving directly to IVF might be more cost-effective than starting with IUI cycles for unexplained and mild male factor infertility.[8] Nevertheless, the balance of published studies still favors starting with IUI before moving to IVF for the treatment of male subfertility. It is time to realize that a better selection of those couples who benefit most from IUI as a first-line treatment is urgently needed and therefore a better understanding of the effect of sperm quality on IUI success is mandatory.

Conclusion

Although our literature search did not reveal Level 1 evidence on the relation between sperm quality and IUI success, a large number of prospective observational studies and well-organized retrospective analyses indicate that above an IMC of 1 million motile spermatozoa, recovered after the washing period is probably the best cost-effective treatment before starting IVF. We urgently need studies to find out which are the cut-off levels of semen parameters above which IUI is an excellent first-line treatment.

TABLE 9.1

Statements of Chapter 9

Statement	Level of Evidence (LOE)
The success rate of IUI is improved with a morphology score of more than 4% normal forms, a TMCS of more than 5 million and an initial total motility of more than 30%	2a
IUI is an acceptable first-line treatment with an IMC of more than 1 million	2a
If the morphology score is more than 4%, IUI can be performed with an acceptable success rate even if the IMC is less than 1 million	3
The influence of sperm parameters on IUI outcome is influenced by other parameters such as female age and number of follicles obtained after ovarian stimulation	3

TABLE 9.2

Recommendations of Chapter 9

Recommendation	Grade Strength
IUI should be used as a first-line treatment in case of moderate male subfertility provided more than 1 million motile spermatozoa are available after washing and at least one tube is patent	B

REFERENCES

1. Tomlinson M. 2010. Is your andrology service up to scratch? *Hum Fertil (Camb)* 13:194–200. Review.
2. Ombelet W., Dhont N., and Kruger T.F. Semen quality and prediction of IUI success: A systematic review. *Reprod Biomed Online*, in press.
3. Van Waart J., Kruger T.F., Lombard C.J., and Ombelet W. 2001. Predictive value of normal sperm morphology in intrauterine insemination (IUI): A structured literature review. *Hum Reprod* 7:495–500.
4. Ombelet W., Deblaere K., Bosmans E., Cox A., Jacobs P., Janssen M., and Nijs M. 2003. Semen quality and intrauterine insemination. *Reprod Biomed Online* 7:485–492.
5. Van Weert J.M., Repping S., Van Voorhis B.J., Van der Veen F., Bossuyt P.M., and Mol B.W. 2004. Performance of the postwash total motile sperm count as a predictor of pregnancy at the time of intrauterine insemination: A meta-analysis. *Fertil Steril* 82:612–620.
6. Ombelet W., Vandeput H., Van de Putte G., Cox A., Janssen M., Jacobs P., Bosmans E., Steeno O., and Kruger T. 1997. Intrauterine insemination after ovarian stimulation with clomiphene citrate: Predictive potential of inseminating motile count and sperm morphology? *Hum Reprod* 12:1458–1463.
7. Van Voorhis B.J., Sparks A.E., Allen B.D., Stovall D.W., Syrop C.H., and Chapler F.K. 1997. Cost-effectiveness of infertility treatments: A cohort study. *Fertil Steril* 67:830–836.
8. Bhatti T. and Baibergenova A. 2008. A comparison of the cost-effectiveness of *in vitro* fertilization strategies and stimulated intrauterine insemination in a Canadian health economic model. *J Obstet Gynaecol Can* 30:411–420.

10

Factors Influencing IUI Outcome: Semen Preparation Techniques

Martine Nijs and Carolien M. Boomsma

Introduction

The human ejaculate consists of the secretions of the accessory glands, the seminal plasma, and spermatozoa. Seminal fluid acts as a transport medium for sperm, providing fructose as an energy source, prostaglandins, and ions such as sodium and potassium, and antioxidants like ascorbic acid or superoxide dismutase. The prostatic secretions are rich in citric acid, zinc, potassium, and choline. Cells other than spermatozoa are also present in the ejaculate, including epithelial cells from the urinary tract, prostate cells, spermatogenic cells, and leukocytes. Reactive oxygen species (ROS), either produced by the different germ cells or by leukocytes, can be detrimental for the fertilizing potential of the spermatozoa.

The semen, more specifically the seminal plasma, contains decapitation factor(s) that need to be removed for complete capacitation of the spermatozoa. This process of capacitation is essential for both fertilization *in vivo* or *in vitro*, and hence spermatozoa to be used in clinical procedures like intra-uterine insemination (IUI) or IVF must be separated from the seminal plasma and its decapacitating factors. This *preparation* or *processing* of the human semen sample should also result in the removal of nonviable spermatozoa, leukocytes, and/or bacteria, elimination of the different secretions, and other sources of contamination from the ejaculate.

Sperm preparation techniques (SPTs) should isolate and select sperm cells with intact functional and genetic properties, including normal morphology, minimal DNA damage, and intact cell membranes with functional binding properties.

In order to improve the quality and outcome of IUI procedures, it is clear that there is a need for simple, inexpensive, reliable, and safe SPTs. This chapter will discuss the scientific evidence that is at present available for defining which SPT to be used and will discuss the practical aspects of these different semen preparations.

Ejaculatory Abstinence, Semen Production, and Transport

Although often neglected, the optimal SPT starts at the time of the production of the ejaculate: correct production, transport, and receipt of the semen sample is essential for good clinical practice and obtaining optimal results.

A clear negative effect of *ejaculatory abstinence time* on sperm quality (WHO parameters) has been demonstrated in multiple studies: a longer abstinence period is associated with higher sperm volume and concentration but sperm motility is lower and sperm DNA fragmentation levels are clearly increased. DNA fragmentation is reduced by implementing short periods of abstinence taking care that it is not shorter than 24 hours, since within-subject analysis demonstrated an increase in poor chromatin packaging with an abstinence period of 24 hours. IUI outcomes were shown to be optimal after 2 days of ejaculatory abstinence.[5] Based on these studies, an abstinence interval of ≤ 2 days is to be advised for patients undergoing IUI.

Semen samples need to be produced in *sterile containers* that have been tested for *reprotoxicity* (some plastics and silicones of the containers can release chemical substances that are negative for sperm viability). The sample needs to be transported to the laboratory *at body temperature* and semen preparation *needs to commence as soon as possible after liquefaction* of the sample: seminal plasma contains several factors that significantly reduce the fertilizing capacity of the spermatozoa after prolonged exposure (≥30 minutes).[4]

Semen Preparation in the Laboratory

Currently, three SPTs for IUI are routinely being used in laboratories worldwide and are described in detail in *The Laboratory Manual for the Examination and Processing of Human Semen of the World Health Organization*.[3] They are the following: simple dilution and washing technique, a sperm separation based on sperm motility or on sperm density, and gravity.

1. *Simple dilution and washing technique*—The simple dilution of semen with a large volume (5 to 10 times) of medium followed by centrifugation (washing) at 300 g for 10 minutes is a basic SPT. The pellet obtained is resuspended in medium and again centrifuged at 300–500 g for 5 minutes, followed by resuspension of the new pellet in a volume of medium appropriate for the insemination and incubation until the time of insemination.

2. *Swim-up technique*—Spermatozoa may be selected by their ability to swim out of seminal plasma and into culture medium, the *swim-up* technique. Morphological abnormal spermatozoa will not be selected out, nor ROS that are present in the semen. This procedure gives a lower yield of spermatozoa than washing and hence is limited to samples with high sperm concentrations. The time allowed for swim up should be adjusted according to the quality of the initial sample: the percentage of abnormal sperm that will appear in the medium increases with time and will continue to do so after normal motile density has reached its optimum level.

   Aliquots of liquefied semen are placed directly under medium (1 ml) in round bottom tubes in order to have the highest medium surface yield. Tubes are placed at at an angle of 45° and incubated up to 1 hour (maximum) at 37°C. The upper part of the layered medium is removed taking care not to disturb the interface and is washed in 2 ml medium (centrifugation at 300–500 g); the final pellet is resuspended and incubated before clinical use.

3. *Density gradient centrifugation* (DGC)—The DGC selects spermatozoa according to their density and gravity (mass per unit volume) and results in cells being dispersed throughout the gradient column according to the gradient that matches their density. Colloidal silica preparations stabilized with covalently bound hydrophilic silane will make an ideal density gradient. Morphologically normal human spermatozoa have a density of 1.12 g/ml; immature abnormal spermatozoa have a density between 1.06 and 1.09 g/ml. Normal spermatozoa can be isolated in the solution with the highest concentration of gradient, which is aspirated for further use. Number and volume of the layers can be adapted according to the initial sperm concentration and percentage of morphological normal spermatozoa.

   A two-layer discontinuous DGC with 1 ml of 40% density top layer over 1 ml of an 80% density medium layer is mostly used. One to 1.5 ml of semen is placed above the gradient column and centrifuged at 300 g for 15 to 20 minutes. The top layer will retain epithelial cells, blood cells, and immature and abnormally shaped sperm cells. The lower layer is removed and resuspended in 5–10 ml of medium and followed by two washing steps at 300 g for 10 minutes. The final pellet is resuspended and incubated before clinical use.

Media to Be Used in IUI

Sperm capacitation requires the presence of bicarbonate ions. If the prepared spermatozoa are to be *stored* after the sperm preparation before the IUI, it is advised to use a *sperm buffer*: a zwitterion-buffered medium (like HEPES). This will avoid premature capacitation and hyperactivated motility during semen preparation and storage (care must be taken that tubes are tightly capped during the storage in the incubator). If the IUI is to be performed soon after sperm processing, *sperm medium*, a bicarbonate-buffered medium, can be used throughout the entire process.

Quality Control and Quality Management in Semen Preparation for IUI

All specimen containers, processing tubes, and pipettes must be labeled according to local guidelines (EU tissue directive 2003) and batches should all be traceable. If no guidelines exist, at least two identifiers (man's name and laboratory reference ID) should be used. Only one specimen is actually worked on at any point in time. Multiple samples may be centrifuged at the same time as long as there is an established procedure for verification of each tube's identity by a witness. All re-identification steps should be documented. The performance of the IUI program should be analyzed regularly: program performance indicators in IUI are recovery rate after SPT, pregnancy and clinical pregnancy rates (broken down by female's age and type of stimulation, and must include the multiple implantation rate). Data should be bench marked against *expected results*, for example, data from literature. Operator performance (laboratory staff and inseminator) is to be evaluated as well.

Evidence for the Use of One SPT Compared to Another

The comparison of different SPTs in relation to semen parameters has been the focus of a substantial amount of research. Most studies evaluate the outcome (WHO parameters)[3] of a semen sample that is split and prepared by the different techniques.

Overall, the DGC is shown to be superior to the swim-up and wash technique: a clear improvement of morphological normal spermatozoa with grade A motility and normal DNA integrity are obtained in the prepared sample. Moreover, ROS and leukocyte concentration is highly reduced when the latter technique is used. Spermatozoa obtained show less chromatin and nuclear DNA anomalies as well as better nuclear maturation rates. Improved acrosome reaction as well as higher hypo-osmotic swelling test reaction occurred after DGC in comparison to the wash or swim-up technique.

The *Cochrane Review* of Boomsma et al.,[1] a meta-analysis, investigated clinical outcomes after IUI in relation to the three different SPTs (wash and centrifugation, swim-up, and DGC) in subfertile couples undergoing IUI. Five randomized controlled trials were included in the meta-analysis with 262 couples in total. The meta-analysis did not show evidence of a difference in the effectiveness of a swim up versus a GDC on pregnancy rates per couple (30.5% versus 21.5% resp; Peto odds ratio 1.57; 95% CI 0.74 to 3.32) (Figure 10.1). Swim-up technique versus wash and centrifugation also showed no significant difference in pregnancy rates (22.2% versus 38.1% resp., Peto odds ratio 0.41, 95% CI 0.15 to 1.10) (Figure 10.2). Two studies compared the gradient versus wash and centrifugation technique with pregnancy rates reaching 23.5% and 13.3%, respectively (Peto odds ratio 1.76, 95% CI 0.57 to 5.44) (Figure 10.3).

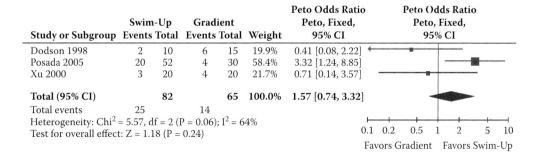

Study or Subgroup	Swim-Up Events	Total	Gradient Events	Total	Weight	Peto Odds Ratio Peto, Fixed, 95% CI	Peto Odds Ratio Peto, Fixed, 95% CI
Dodson 1998	2	10	6	15	19.9%	0.41 [0.08, 2.22]	
Posada 2005	20	52	4	30	58.4%	3.32 [1.24, 8.85]	
Xu 2000	3	20	4	20	21.7%	0.71 [0.14, 3.57]	
Total (95% CI)		**82**		**65**	**100.0%**	**1.57 [0.74, 3.32]**	
Total events	25		14				

Heterogeneity: Chi^2 = 5.57, df = 2 (P = 0.06); I^2 = 64%
Test for overall effect: Z = 1.18 (P = 0.24)

0.1 0.2 0.5 1 2 5 10
Favors Gradient   Favors Swim-Up

FIGURE 10.1 Swim-up versus gradient technique. A comparison of pregnancy rates per couple.

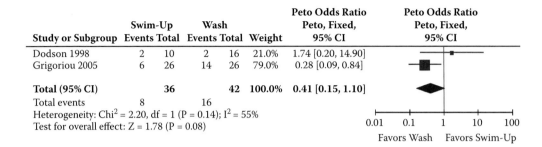

FIGURE 10.2 Swim-up versus wash technique. A comparison of pregnancy rates per couple.

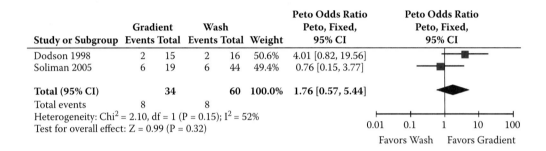

FIGURE 10.3 Gradient versus wash technique. A comparison of pregnancy rates per couple.

Overall, there was no clear evidence of which SPT was superior. The authors concluded that there is insufficient evidence to recommend any specific SPT on the basis of these RCTs. Large, high quality randomized controlled trials comparing the effectiveness of GDC, swim up and wash, and centrifugation technique on clinical outcomes are lacking but are warranted.[1]

Selecting Your SPT

Each ART unit should make their proper evaluation of the usefulness and applicability of any SPT by comparing the quantitative (relative and absolute yield of progressive motile spermatozoa obtained) and qualitative aspects (pregnancy ratio) as well as the practicalities (simplicity, costs in materials, and rapidity in laboratory costs) of each SPT.

The WHO laboratory manual[3] suggests the choice of the type of SPT is dictated by the nature of the semen sample. Swim up generally produces a lower recovery of motile spermatozoa (<20%) than does DGC (>20%) (see Table 10.1).

Novel Developments of Sperm Selection Methods

Several novel sperm selection methods have recently been developed for IVF and ICSI. These methods aim at isolating mature, structurally intact, and nonapoptotic spermatozoa with high DNA integrity (review by Said and Land[2]). Their value in IUI sperm preparation still needs to be demonstrated (see Table 10.2).

Selection Based on Sperm Surface Charge

An electrophoresis-based technology has been developed to separate spermatozoa based on size and electronegative charge. The latter indicates that the sperm is normally differentiated and expresses CD52 (a specific surface protein), which was found to be correlated with normal sperm morphology and capacitation. This technique may be considered for samples with high DNA damage since it is capable of selecting sperm with intact DNA. Unfortunately, the technique did not show improved fertilization rates nor improved embryo quality in ICSI.[2]

The Zeta method selects sperm with respect to membrane surface charges or Zeta potential. Washed sperm is pipetted into a positively charged centrifuge and centrifuged. Thereafter, adhering (negatively charged, mature) sperm can be retrieved by rinsing the tube. The Zeta method tended to increase fertilization, implantation, and pregnancy rates.[2]

Nonapoptotic Sperm Selection

Magnetic cell sorting (MACS) using annexin-V microbeads can effectively separate apoptotic and non-apoptotic spermatozoa, as apoptotic cells present phospholipid phosphatidylserine on the outer sperm

TABLE 10.1

Statements of Chapter 10

Statement	Level of Evidence (LOE)
SPTs significantly increased the probability of conception after IUI in couples with male subfertility	1b
ROS can be detrimental for the fertilizing potential of the spermatozoa	2b
IUI outcomes showed to be optimal after 2 days of ejaculatory abstinence	2a
The sample needs to be transported to the laboratory at body temperature	2b
Semen samples need to be produced in sterile containers that have been tested for reprotoxicity	2a
Semen preparation needs to commence as soon as possible after liquefaction of the sample	2b
If the prepared spermatozoa are to be *stored* after the sperm preparation before the IUI, it is advised to use a *sperm buffer* (e.g., HEPES medium)	3
If the IUI is to be performed soon after sperm processing, a bicarbonate buffered-medium can be used throughout the entire process	3
Concerning laboratory outcomes (e.g., semen parameters): the DGC is shown to be superior to the swim-up and wash technique (improvement of morphological normal spermatozoa with grade A motility and normal DNA integrity, reduced concentrations of ROS and leukocytes, less chromatin and nuclear DNA anomalies, better nuclear maturation rates, improved acrosome reaction, and higher hypo-osmotic swelling test reaction)	2a
Concerning clinical outcome (pregnancy rates) after IUI: there is no clear evidence of which SPT is superior	1a
Selection based on sperm surface charge did not lead to any improvement in fertilization rates or embryo quality following ICSI. The Zeta potential method was reported in one study to increase fertilization, implantation, and pregnancy rates, although not significant	2a
Nonapoptotic sperm selection by MACS resulted in spermatozoa with higher motility and less apoptosis, higher embryo cleavage, and higher pregnancy rates. Fertilization or implantation rates were not higher.	2a

TABLE 10.2

Recommendations of Chapter 10

Recommendation	Grade Strength
Quality control and quality management in semen preparation for IUI is mandatory	GPP
Clinical outcome after IUI: there is insufficient evidence to recommend any specific SPT	A
Laboratory outcomes: the DGC is shown to be superior to the swim-up and wash technique	B
Novel sperm selection methods (based on sperm surface charge or nonapoptotic sperm selection) show promising results. However, they have not yet established themselves in routine practice, and their purpose for IUI is unknown; more evidence is needed	D

surface that will bind to the magnetic microbeads. The selection of nonapoptotic spermatozoa by MACS resulted in an enriched nonapoptotic, motile sperm population; higher embryo cleavage and pregnancy rates were obtained. Neither fertilization nor implantation rates, however, were improved.[2]

REFERENCES

1. Boomsma C.M., Heineman M.J., Cohlen B.J., and Farquhar C. 2012. Semen preparation techniques for intrauterine insemination. *Cochrane Database Syst Revs* 6.
2. Said T.M. and Land J.A. 2011. Effects of advanced selection methods on sperm quality and ART outcome: A systematic review. *Hum Reprod Update* 17:719–733.
3. World Health Organization. 2010. *WHO Laboratory Manual for the Examination and Processing of Human Semen*, 5th ed. Geneva: WHO Press.
4. Bjorndahl L., Mortimer D., Barratt C., Castilla J.A., Menkveld R., and Kvist U. 2010. *A Practical Guide to Basic Laboratory Andrology*. Cambridge: Cambridge University Press.
5. Nijs M. 2009. *Study of Sperm Parameters in Assisted Reproduction Outcome*. Maastricht, The Netherlands: Datawyse Boekproducties.

11

Factors Influencing IUI Outcome: Time Interval as a Prognostic Factor

Roberto Matorras, Olga Ramón, Beatriz Corcostegui, Lorena Crisol, and Antonia Exposito

Introduction

A number of studies have shown how a wide range of environmental factors can have a detrimental effect on oocytes and embryos including exposure to light, temperatures beyond certain ranges, polyvinyl chloride, and polychlorinated biphenyls, as well as other environmental conditions.[2] Indeed, the importance of keeping embryo temperature close to 37°C and O_2 and CO_2 concentrations within specific ranges is well known and a number of technological devices have been designed to avoid fluctuations in these conditions for oocytes and embryos during their manipulation and storage. Moreover, in ICSI cycles it is well known that the success of the procedure is clearly related to the learning curve of the embryologist: the longer the time spent on the insemination, the poorer the result. Similarly, we have shown how the time interval between embryo catheter loading and discharging influences the success of IVF: the longer the interval, the poorer the results.[2]

Concerning sperm, the 5th edition of the WHO semen manual recommends that semen samples be collected in a private room near the laboratory, in order to limit the exposure of the semen to fluctuations in temperature and to limit the time between collection and analysis. It is underlined that the semen sample should be delivered to the laboratory within 1 hour of collection.

On the other hand, although sperm progressive motility of a freshly ejaculated semen specimen declines both over time and with exposure to extremes of temperature, it is also known that a freshly ejaculated semen specimen will maintain an acceptable sperm progressive motility for up to 12 hours, and spermatozoa will survive up to 24 to 48 hours. There is considerable experience showing that if the semen sample is not exposed to extreme temperatures and is delivered to the laboratory within 1 hour of collection, there is no notable influence on sperm parameters. However, the parameters used to characterize sperm may not accurately reflect the sperm fertilizing ability. Notwithstanding, this 1-hour period, validated only in the diagnostic context, has been systematically applied in the clinical setting without further research.

In the present work, we review the existing evidence in intra-uterine insemination (IUI) cycles on the influence of the times taken for each of the different steps between ejaculation and insemination.

Material and Methods (Table 11.3)

Until now, four series have been reported analyzing the influence of the duration of the different steps in the procedure on IUI results. None of the aforementioned studies was randomized. Two of them are described in journal articles[6,7] and two in congress abstracts.[3,4] An additional abstract was excluded from this analysis, since the results were reported in a later paper that has been included.[7] Three of the papers were written in English[4,6,7] and the other one in Spanish.[3]

In two of them no significant differences were observed,[3,6] whereas the other two studies[4,7] reported shorter intervals among women achieving pregnancy. Concerning ovarian stimulation, in two series, ovarian stimulation was performed with FSH,[3,4] either gonadotrophins or clomiphene citrate being used in the others.[6,7] In one of the studies, hMG and clomiphene data were reported separately,[7] and we have considered them independently. A further difference was that in two cases the semen samples were obtained at the hospital,[3,4] while in the others the collection was either at the hospital or at home.[6,7] Since the influence of the time elapsing could be different in the different steps of the IUI procedures, besides analyzing the total time spent on the procedure, that is from ejaculation to insemination (collection-insemination interval), two additional periods were considered: the time elapsing between the ejaculation and the beginning of preparation (collection-preparation interval) and the time between the preparation and the insemination. The time spent on sperm processing was assumed to be constant and was not considered in any of the aforementioned studies.[3,4,6,7] In one study, the collection-insemination and preparation-insemination intervals had a very similar duration,[6] while in two the collection-insemination interval was almost twice as long as the preparation-insemination interval,[3,4] and in the fourth study the reverse was true.[7]

A very recent paper[1] studied only the influence of the interval between sperm wash and IUI and pregnancy rates. It was not included in the meta-analysis, since no data were given concerning mean intervals in cycles achieving pregnancy and nonachieving pregnancy.

Results (Table 11.4)

Collection-Insemination (CI) Interval

Reported mean CI intervals ranged from 70 to 156 minutes.[6,7] In the smaller two series[4,7] pregnancy was associated with shorter CI intervals (99 ± 7 versus 156 ± 13 and 134.2 ± 23.8 versus 145.5 ± 24.7) while there were no significant differences in the larger series (139.9 ± 25.3 versus 128.0 ± 25.8 and 70 ± 19 versus 73 ± 18).[3,6] Notably, when the results were combined, the mean values were almost identical (100.7 ± 21.2 versus 96.9 ± 20.2), without significant differences.

Collection-Preparation (CP) Interval

Reported mean CP intervals ranged from 20 to 76.1 minutes.[4,6] Pregnancy was associated with shorter CI intervals in the smaller two series (27 ± 4 versus 41 ± 3 and 61.4 ± 26.3 versus 76.1 ± 20.7)[4,7] while there were no significant differences in the larger series (20 ± 11 versus 20 ± 13 and 49.3 ± 17.3 versus 47.8 ± 16.9).[3,6] When the results were combined, the mean values were very similar in couples achieving pregnancy (33.5 ± 14.7) and in those nonachieving pregnancy (31.5 ± 13.4), without significant differences.

Preparation-Insemination (PI) Interval

There was also a wide range in PI intervals, mean values ranging from 18 to 85 minutes.[6,7] A significantly longer PI interval among women not reaching pregnancy was reported only in the hMG-treated subset of one series (42 ± 5 versus 85 ± 12).[7] There were no significant differences between the PI interval in couples achieving and not achieving pregnancy in any of the other series. When the results were combined, the mean values were very similar in couples achieving pregnancy (24.1 ± 14.4) and in those nonachieving pregnancy (26.5 ± 13.3), without significant differences.

Conclusions

There is a paucity of studies on the influence of the time elapsing between semen collection and the insemination on IUI results. The first paper on the topic reported an impairment in pregnancy rates in hMG cycles when the CP interval was prolonged.[7] This finding could be explained by some changes reported in sperm after collection: prolonged exposure to spermatozoa decapacitation and reactive oxygen species, exhaustion of energy sources, increase in sperm DNA fragmentation, or encephalin levels. On the other hand, it has been proposed that sperm washing could be performed at home by the same couple, allowing it to incubate for 2 hours prior to IUI during transport.[5] This allowed patients to collect IUI specimens in the comfort and privacy of their home.

As far as we know, only four previous studies have been conducted analyzing the influence of time intervals on insemination results; of these, only two have been published in journals and none of the studies were randomized. Among the aforementioned studies there was remarkable heterogeneity concerning methodology and cycle management, as well as the times spent on the different steps of IUI. Moreover, while significant differences were found in the two smaller studies,[4,7] no differences were detected in the larger studies.[3,6]

Further, various sources of bias could not be ruled out: for instance, prolonged times between collection and preparation could be associated with older men, and this could be responsible for the poorer results (either directly the effect of the man's age itself or by the associated older age of the woman). We are also unable to rule out that in couples knowing that they had a poor prognosis, the collection-preparation interval could be lengthened by psychological factors, and the lower pregnancy rates could then be attributable to the previously known poor prognosis.

In a very recent paper[1] analyzing only the PI interval, not included in our meta-analysis because of lacking mean values in pregnant and nonpregnant cases, even somewhat lower pregnancy rates were reported when the PI interval was <30 minutes.

In the meta-analysis we performed, mean times were very similar in the different insemination steps in women who did and did not become pregnant. Only in the small series was a significantly reduced CP interval associated with pregnancy. Overall, the differences observed do not seem to be related to the different time intervals reported in the different works.

TABLE 11.3

Characteristics of the Included Studies

First Author	Yavas	Song	Meabe	Ramon
Year	2004	2007	2008	2011
Patients	62	335	152	38
Cycles	132	633	305	50
Stimulation	Clomiphene (95) or hMG (37)	Clomiphene hMG or FSH	FSH	FSH
Place of sperm collection	Home (95) Clinic (37)	Home (236) Clinic (3971)	Hospital	Hospital
Pregnancy rates	8.2% (6/73) (Clomiphene) 27% (10/37) (hMG)	13.9% (88/633)	17% (56/305)	28% (14/50)

TABLE 11.4

Meta-Analysis

	Collection–Preparation		Preparation–Insemination		Collection–Insemination	
	Pregnancy	No Pregnancy	Pregnancy	No Pregnancy	Pregnancy	No Pregnancy
Yavas (CC)	28 ± 4	38 ± 2	51 ± 11	63.8 ± 8	109 ± 14	131 ± 9
Yavas (hMG)	27 ± 4*	41 ± 3	42 ± 5*	85 ± 12	99 ± 7*	156 ± 13
Song	20 ± 11	20 ± 13	18 ± 12	20 ± 13	70 ± 19	73 ± 18
Meabe	49.3 ± 17.3	47.75 ± 16.9	27.4 ± 18.5	26.0 ± 15.1	139.9 ± 25.3	128.0 ± 25.8
Ramón	61.4 ± 26.3*	76.1 ± 20.7	27.8 ± 13.2	24.3 ± 14.2	134.2 ± 23.8*	145.5 ± 24.8
Total	33.5 ± 14.7	31.5 ± 13.4	24.1 ± 14.4	26.5 ± 13.3	100.7 ± 21.2	96.9 ± 20.2

*p < 0.05.
No significant differences in the meta-analysis results.

TABLE 11.1

Statements of Chapter 11

Statement	Level of Evidence (LOE)
There is no evidence that shorter intervals for the various steps of IUI (collection-preparation; preparation-insemination; and collection-insemination) are associated with a better prognosis	2a
There have been no randomized studies on this topic	1

TABLE 11.2

Recommendations of Chapter 11

Recommendation	Grade Strength
More research is needed to investigate the importance of the time interval in IUI results	C
Since reducing intervals is inexpensive and risk-free, we recommend that times associated with IUI procedure are reduced, especially the interval between sperm collection and processing, which should be less than 60 min, preferably less than 45 min (LOE 3)	C

From our analysis, we conclude that there is no evidence that—in the ranges considered in the studies available—prolonged intervals between sperm collection and preparation, between sperm preparation and insemination, or overall from sperm collection to insemination have a detrimental effect on insemination results (see also Tables 11.1 and 11.2).

Notwithstanding the aforementioned criticisms, some of the available data suggests that IUI success rates could be affected by the length of these intervals in some specific contexts. In the ranges studied, the step in which it would perhaps be beneficial to avoid delays is that from collection to preparation, whereas the preparation-insemination interval does not seem to be time dependent, at least in the ranges considered in these studies.

REFERENCES

1. Kilicdag E.B. 2012. The effect of intervals from sperm wash to intra uterine insemination (IUI) time on pregnancy rate. *J Turk Soc Obstet Gynecol* 9:159–63.
2. Matorras R., Mendoza R., Expósito A., and Rodriguez-Escudero F.J. 2004. Influence of the time interval between embryo catheter loading and discharging on the success of IVF. *Hum Reprod* 19:2027–30.
3. Meabe A., Cobos P., Abanto E., Burgos J., Corcostegui B., and Ramón O. 2008. Influence of Time in Intrauterine Insemination Results. 27th Meeting of the Spanish Infertility Society. Oviedo, Spain, May 20–25, 2008.
4. Ramón O., Corcostegui B., Crisol L., Exposito A., Múgica J., and Matorras R. 2011. Sperm Processing: The Time Interval as Prognostic Factor in Intrauterine Insemination (IUI). 27th Annual Meeting of the ESHRE. Stockholm, Sweden, July 3–7, 2011.
5. Randall G.W. and Gantt P.A. 2007. Intrauterine insemination results in couples requiring extended semen transport time. *Int J Fertil Womens Med* 52:28–34.
6. Song G.J., Herko R., and Lewis V. 2007. Location of semen collection and time interval from collection to use for intrauterine insemination. *Fertil Steril* 88:1689–91.
7. Yavas Y. and Selub M.R. 2004. Intrauterine insemination (IUI) pregnancy outcome is enhanced by shorter intervals from semen collection to sperm wash, from sperm wash to IUI time, and from semen collection to IUI time. *Fertil Steril* 82:1638–47.

12

Factors Influencing IUI Outcome: Number of Cycles to Perform

Inge M. Custers

When homologous intra-uterine insemination (IUI) is commenced, information on the optimum number of cycles to perform is essential. Unfortunately, exact data on the optimum number of cycles, as a possible limit to which IUI is effective, is lacking. Advice on the optimum number of cycles to perform vary between three to 12 cycles in the literature.[1–9]

Several randomized studies have shown that IUI without mild ovarian hyperstimulation increases the chance of pregnancy up to six treatment cycles. This effect is seen in all diagnoses for which IUI is applied: mild male factor, cervical factor, unexplained subfertility, and mild (stage I and II) endometriosis.[2,5,8] At the same time, pregnancy chances per cycle decrease after every attempt.[10] In several randomized and nonrandomized studies it was confirmed that the majority of pregnancies occur in the first three cycles, so the largest chance of an ongoing pregnancy per cycle is in the first three attempts.[1–4] Evidence on the effectiveness of IUI after the sixth cycle is limited, only a minor number of studies have investigated the effect of repeating IUI after six attempts in large cohorts; these studies were all retrospective cohort studies.[3,4] The largest multi-center study consisted of 3,714 patients of which 430 couples continued treatment after six previous failed attempts. After six cycles of IUI the cumulative ongoing pregnancy rate was found to be 30% and after nine completed cycles 41%. The authors concluded that pregnancy chances per cycle significantly dropped after the first three cycles (OR for an ongoing pregnancy in the third treatment cycle compared to the first cycle 0.68; 95% CI 0.55–0.84) but remain fairly stable from the sixth up to the ninth treatment cycle (ORs for sixth and ninth cycle compared to the first cycle 0.62; 95% CI 0.47–0.82 and 0.61; 95% CI 0.25–1.50).

From these data it was suggested that if time is not an issue some couples could be offered nine treatment cycles, especially couples in which the female age is below 35 years.[4]

In conclusion, patients receiving IUI with or without ovarian stimulation should be offered preferably six treatment cycles. An absolute minimum of treatment cycles that should be offered is three, and if time is not an issue, some patients (especially young women below 35 years of age) can continue IUI until a maximum of nine cycles (see Tables 12.1 and 12.2).

TABLE 12.1

Statements of Chapter 12

Statement	Level of Evidence (LOE)
The pregnancy rate per cycle is highest in the first three treatment cycles	1b
Couples with mild male subfertility, unexplained fertility problems, or mild endometrioses show acceptable cumulative ongoing pregnancy rates after six cycles of IUI with OH	1b
After the third treatment cycle, ongoing pregnancy rates per cycle remain stable up to the ninth treatment cycle	2a

TABLE 12.2

Recommendations of Chapter 12

Recommendation	Grade Strength
Couples with mild male subfertility, unexplained fertility problems, or mild endometrioses should be offered six cycles of IUI	A
Three cycles of IUI is the absolute minimum that should be offered	B
Young couples (below 35 years of age) should be offered the possibility to continue IUI up to nine cycles	B

REFERENCES

1. Aboulghar M., Mansour R., Serour G., Abdrazek A. et al. 2001. Controlled ovarian hyperstimulation and intrauterine insemination for treatment of unexplained infertility should be limited to a maximum of three trials. *Fertil Steril* 75(1):88–91.
2. Bensdorp A., Cohlen B.J., Heineman M.J., and Vanderkerchove P. 2009. Intra-uterine insemination for male subfertility. *Cochrane Database Sys Rev.* doi: 10.1002/14651858.CD000360.pub4.
3. Berg U., Brucker C., Berg F.D. 1997. Effect of motile sperm count after swim-up on outcome of intra-uterine insemination. *Fertil Steril* 67(4):747–750.
4. Custers I.M., Steures P., Hompes P., Flierman P. et al. 2008. Intrauterine insemination: How many cycles should we perform? *Hum Reprod* 23(4):885–888.
5. Goverde A.J., McDonnel J., Vermeiden J.P.W., Schats R. et al. 2000. Intrauterine insemination or *in vitro* fertilisation in idiopathic subfertility: A randomised trial and cost-effectiveness analysis. *Lancet* January 355 (9197):13–18.
6. Merviel P., Heraud M.H., Grenier N., Lourdel E. et al. 2010. Predictive factors for pregnancy after intrauterine insemination (IUI): An analysis of 1038 cycles and a review of the literature. *Fertil Steril* 93(1):79–88.
7. Papageorgiou T.C., Guibert J., Savale M., Goffinet F. et al. 2004. Low dose recombinant FSH treatment may reduce multiple gestations caused by controlled ovarian hyperstimulation and intrauterine insemination. *BJOG* 111:1277–1282.
8. Reindollar R.H., Regan M.M., Neumann P.J., Levine B.S. et al, 2010. A randomized clinical trial to evaluate optimal treatment for unexplained subfertility: The fast track and standard treatment (FASTT) trial. *Fertil Steril* 94(3):888–899.
9. Sahakyan M., Harlow B.L., and Hornstein M.D. 1999. Influence of age, diagnosis and cycle number on pregnancy rates with gonadotrophin-induced controlled ovarian hyperstimulation and intrauterine insemination. *Fertil Steril* 72(3):500–504.
10. Steures P. and Van der Steeg J.W. for CECERM. 2004. Prediction of an ongoing pregnancy after intra-uterine insemination. *Fertil Steril* 82(1):45–51.

13

Factors Influencing IUI Outcome: Perifollicular Flow and Endometrial Thickness

Geeta Nargund, Vasileios Sarafis, and Stuart Campbell

The aim of intra-uterine insemination (IUI) is to enable a mature oocyte from the woman and spermatozoa from her partner to be brought in close proximity to maximize the chances of fertilization and implantation. This implies that the tubes are patent, the endometrium is receptive, and the egg and sperm are of good quality. This chapter will assess how ultrasound can be used to provide important information on egg quality and endometrial receptivity that will optimize the chances of success. This qualitative information requires the addition of Doppler assessment of ovarian and endometrial angiogenesisis to the basic 2D ultrasound examination.

Doppler Ultrasound

Doppler ultrasound measures the change of frequency caused by movement in tissues and is particularly useful in assessing the movement of red blood cells in blood vessels and capillaries. There are several methods of displaying and measuring Doppler signals. Spectral Doppler has been used for many years to measure the velocity of flow in blood vessels. To measure absolute velocity (in cm/sec) the vessels are first displayed as a color Doppler map on the 2D ultrasound image, a "gate" is placed over the vessel of interest and a flow velocity waveform obtained. To measure peak systolic velocity (PSV) accurately, corrections have to be made for the angle between the Doppler beam and the blood vessel. With small angiogenic vessels which show on the color Doppler map as a network of color signals, angle correction is not required as these vessels travel in different directions and as many of these will be included in the Doppler gate, PSV measurement is reproducible. Other parameters that can be measured with spectral Doppler are the impedance indices like pulsatility index (PI) and resistance index (RI). These measure the resistance to flow by providing a ratio between systolic and diastolic velocities and have the advantage if being angle independent. A reduction of PI implies an increase in blood flow. Recently, there has been an emphasis on the visualization of vascularity by means of power Doppler ultrasound which provides a two-dimensional map of Doppler signals superimposed on the 2D image. This map represents the power of the Doppler signals and in most studies they have been subjectively quantified to assess the amount and intensity of flow in an area of angiogenesis. Most basic ultrasound machines have now been equipped to perform these Doppler assessments. More expensive machines with 3D capability can measure 3D flow indices, that is, the vascularity index (VI) and flow index (FI) to determine the amount and intensity of flow in a 3D volume of the region of interest. However, these measurements are outside the brief of this chapter and the value of these indices has yet to be determined. Many centers now focus on power Doppler assessment of flow rather than spectral Doppler in gynecology. It should be stressed, however, that both these parameters are measuring different things; one is measuring the velocity of flow from arteries in a vessel or localized area of angiogenesis; the other is measuring intensity of flow in a region from both arteries and veins. Both contribute to our knowledge of angiogenesis in the ovary, follicle, and endometrium.

Oocyte Quality

The standard clinical criteria used to assess the quality and maturity of the oocyte is the size of the follicular diameter (or volume) of the dominant follicle(s) on a TV scan and serum estradiol levels. Doppler ultrasound, however, has the potential to give additional valuable information on intrafollicular events that should permit better timing of IUI and consequently improved results. The rapid development of the theca and its vascular network during secondary oocyte development is essential for oocyte competence. It has been shown from studies on IVF stimulated ovaries that blood flow in the capillary network in the theca interna varies between different follicles and that follicles with poor vascularity are associated with low dissolved oxygen content, low PI, and malformed meiotic spindles in the oocyte.[1,2] Studies using color Doppler have shown that perifollicular vascularity can be visualized from the middle of the follicular phase but the intensity of color signals and the spectral velocities increase dramatically after the LH surge (Figure 13.1). Nargund et al.[3] demonstrated that at the time of egg collection in IVF cycles, the probability of producing an oocyte that progressed to grade I or grade II embryo was 70% if the perifollicular PSV was >10 cm/sec. while absence of flow was associated in over 80% of cases with a poor quality embryo or no embryo at all. Similar results were found when studies were repeated before hCG administration indicating that perifollicular PSV could be used to alter clinical management.[4] This group found that the PI of flow from perifollicular vessels was not helpful in predicting outcome although the values were invariably <1 indicating that angiogenic vessels have low resistance flow. Power Doppler studies have also been used to grade follicles as to their potential in producing a fertilizable oocyte. Most studies have used the four categories of flow described by Bhal et al.[5] in which the follicle circumference is divided into quarters of visualized flow, less than 25% being grade 1 (poor vascularization) and more than 75% being grade 4 (high vascularization). This group found that in 181 women undergoing stimulated IUI cycles the two independent variables that affected pregnancy rates were serum estradiol and high-grade perifollicular flow. Using the same methodology these findings were confirmed by other workers in IVF cycles. Robson et al.[6] found a significant trend to higher pregnancy rates when the embryo transfer cohort contained at least one oocyte from a highly vascularized follicle while Monteleone et al.[7] reported that highly vascularized follicles were associated with a higher rate of fertilization and higher pregnancy rates. In the latter study, intrafollicular VEGF levels were significantly correlated with the grade of perifollicular vascularity.

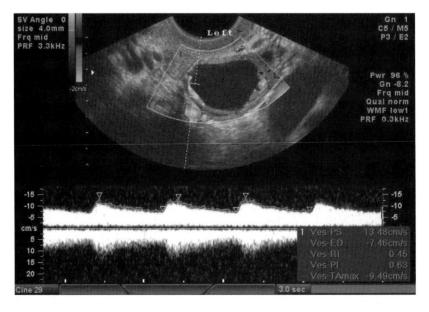

FIGURE 13.1   Perifollicular blood flow in a pre-ovulatory follicle. A gate is correctly placed over the perifollicular vessels. The PSV is 13.5 cm/sec indicating imminent ovulation and a high chance of oocyte competence.

Thus, there is a large body of literature that confirms that oocyte competence is related to perifollicular vascularity as assessed by either spectral Doppler measurements of PSV or subjective assessment of power Doppler signals around the circumference of the follicle. Not all studies have shown a correlation between perifollicular vascularity and the quality of the embryo or pregnancy rates but the overwhelming mass of evidence indicates that this is a clinically important measure of oocyte competence. For the less experienced doctor, subjective power Doppler assessments are easier to make than spectral perifollicular PSV measurements. Failure to detect perifollicular vascularity during IUI treatment should raise suspicion that the follicle is immature or the oocyte incompetent. Delay in giving hCG may result in improvement but if vascularity does not improve then the likelihood of obtaining a competent oocyte from the follicle is significantly reduced. The clinical implications would be to decide if a cycle should be canceled or continued based on vascularity and also to predict the risk of multiple pregnancy if more than one follicle is well vascularized in stimulated cycles.

Endometrial Receptivity

Failure of an adequate endometrial response in the presence of an apparently normally developing follicle and rising estradiol levels indicates that the problem probably lies at the endometrial level. The standard ultrasound criteria of endometrial receptivity are the measurement of endometrial thickness (ET) and endometrial morphology. Bakos et al.[8] described the cyclical changes in the endometrium in 23 healthy volunteers. With the LH peak designated as day 0, the classical hypoechoic triple layer of proliferative endometrium was visible on day −6 with increasing hypoechoic appearance and progressive thickening occurring until at ovulation the mean thickness was 12.4 mm (range 10.0–15.9) (Figure 13.2). From days +1 to +6, increasing echogenicity and blurring between the lines became apparent. In a large study of over 1,000 infertile women, De Geyter et al.[9] found endometrial thickness at the time of spontaneous LH surge (or hCG administration) was significantly lower in untreated women and those receiving short protocol IUI than patients receiving IVF treatment, the figures for mean ET being 9.88 mm, 10.34 mm, and 11.46 mm, respectively, in the three groups. ET did not correlate with the age of the patient but did correlate significantly with estradiol levels on the day of hCG administration. In patients receiving IUI treatment, pregnancy rates were significantly lower when the ET was less than 6.3 mm but there was no minimal thickness for ET in

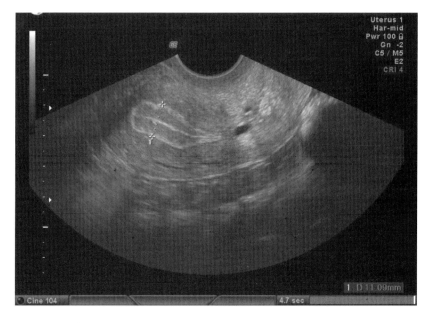

FIGURE 13.2   Typical triple layer endometrium in the preovulatory phase.

patients receiving IVF/ICSI. In fact, the pregnancy rates in this latter group were slightly higher in association with a thinner ET suggesting that higher estradiol levels may not favor implantation. Most studies carried out in IVF cycles have found no overall correlation between ET and pregnancy rates but several groups have found a minimal thickness below which implantation is severely reduced. For example, Khalifa et al.[10] reported a minimal endometrial thickness of 7 mm below, which there is suboptimal implantation.

Endometrial morphology is also of importance in predicting endometrial receptivity. Classification of the appearance of the endometrium has been simplified in recent years and nowadays the endometrium is described as multi-layered (or hypoechoic triple layer) or non-multilayered (or echogenic homogeneous). Serafini et al.[11] found a significantly higher pregnancy rate per ET for women with a hypoechoic multilayered endometrium in the late proliferative phase as compared with women with a homogeneous hyperechoic pattern and several groups have confirmed these findings. It should be stressed that about 5% of patients will have an abnormal endometrium due to endometrial pathology. For example, patients with a thick hyperechoic endometrium may have an endometrial polyp and some with a thin or irregular endometrium at the time of ovulation may have intracavitary adhesions.

Two Doppler techniques have proved useful in predicting implantation. Spectral Doppler studies[12] of the uterine arteries at the time of hCG administration in IVF cycles has shown lower implantation rates in women with a PI >3. Power Doppler studies of the subendometrial vascularity[13] have shown higher implantation rates when the spiral artery flow can be visualized penetrating into the hypoechoic area of the triple layer endometrium (Figure 13.3). These studies can be performed with basic ultrasound equipment and can modify the timing of hCG injection if the Doppler results are suboptimal.

In summary, endometrial thickness in stimulated IUI cycles is lower than in IVF cycles and is lower in cycles stimulated with clompihene citrate than in normal natural cycles.[14] There is no correlation between endometrial thickness and pregnancy rate although an ET less than 6 mm indicates a lower chance of implantation. Persistently thick echogenic endometrium in the follicular phase requires hysteroscopy and biopsy or removal of a polyp if present. Persistently thin or irregular endometrium can be associated with intracavitary adhesions (see Tables 13.1 and 13.2).

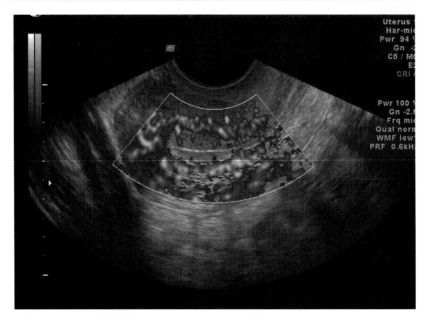

FIGURE 13.3 Power Doppler image showing strong signals from the spiral arteries. The vessels are seen to invade the triple layer.

TABLE 13.1

Statements of Chapter 13

Statement	Level of Evidence (LOE)
Perifollicular blood flow correlates with the maturity of each follicle	2
Perifollicular flow velocity (PSV) above 10 cm/sec or visualization of power Doppler flow more than ¾ around the circumference of the follicle increases the probability of there being a good quality egg following hCG or LH surge	2
Endometrial thickness reflects estrogen levels produced by growing follicle(s)	1
There is no correlation between endometrial thickness and pregnancy rate but an ET less than 6.3 mm is associated with poor receptivity	2
Triple layer endometrial morphology with spiral artery invasion of the endometrium on power Doppler is more predictive of pregnancy than endometrial thickness alone	3

TABLE 13.2

Recommendations of Chapter 13

Recommendation	Grade Strength
In an IUI cycle, if there is poor perifollicular flow (<3 cm/sec) when the follicle is mature, consideration should be given to canceling the cycle	C
If more than three follicles have strong perifollicular flow (>10 cm/sec), IUI should be canceled because of high risk of multiple pregnancy	GPP
A thick echogenic endometrium or a thin irregular endometrium before LH surge or hCG administration is an indication for hysteroscopy	A

REFERENCES

1. Gaulden M. 1992. The enigma of Down syndrome and other trisomic conditions. *Mutation Res* 269:68–88.
2. Van Blerkom J. and Henry G. 1992. Oocyte dysmorphism and aneuploidy in meiotically-mature human oocytes after controlled ovarian stimulation. *Hum Reprod* 7:379–390.
3. Nargund G., Bourne T., Doyle P. et al. 1996. Associations between ultrasound indices of follicular blood flow, oocyte recovery and preimplantation embryo quality. *Hum Reprod* 11:109–113.
4. Nargund G., Doyle P., Bourne T. et al. 1996. Ultrasound derived indices of follicular blood flow before HCG administration and the prediction of oocyte recovery and preimplantation embryo quality. *Hum Reprod* 11:2515–2517.
5. Bhal P.S., Pugh N.D., Gregory L. et al. 2001. Perifollicularity vascularity as a potential variable affecting outcome in stimulated intrauterine insemination treatment cycles: A study using transvaginal power Doppler. *Hum Reprod* 16:1682–1689.
6. Robson S.J., Barry M., and Norman R.J. 2008. Power Doppler assessment of follicle vascularity at the time of oocyte retrieval in *in vitro* fertilization cycles. *Fert Steril* 90:2179–2182.
7. Monteleone P., Artini P.G., Simi G. et al. 2008. Follicular fluid levels directly correlate with perifollicular blood flow in normoresponder patients undergoing IVF. *J. Assist Reprod Genet* 25:183–186.
8. Bakos O., Lundkvist O., and Bergh T. 1993. Transvaginal sonographic evaluation of endometrial growth and texture in spontaneous ovulatory cycles—A descriptive study. *Hum Reprod* 8:799–806.
9. De Geyter C., Schmitter M., De Geyter M. et al. 2000. Prospective evaluation of the ultrasound appearance of the endometrium in a cohort of 1,186 infertile women. *Fert Steril* 73:106–113.
10. Khalifa E., Brzvski R.G., Oehninger S. et al. 1992. Sonographic appearance of the endometrium: The predictive value for the outcome of *in vitro* fertilisation in stimulated cycles. *Hum Reprod* 7:677–680.
11. Serafini P., Batzofin J., Nelson J. et al. 1994. Sonographic uterine predictors of pregnancy in women undergoing ovulation induction for assisted reproductive treatments. *Fertil Steril* 62:815–822.
12. Zaidi J., Campbell S., Pittrof R., Tan S.L. 1995. Endometrial thickness, morphology, vascular penetration and velocimetry in predicting implantation in an *in vitro* fertilization program. *Ultrasound Obstet Gynecol* 6:191–198.

13. Zaidi, J., Pittrof, R., Shaker, A, Kyei-Mensah, A., Campbell, S. and Tan, S.L. 1996. Assessment of uterine artery blood flow on the day of human chorionic gonadotrophin administration by transvaginal color doppler ultrasound in an *in vitro* fertilization program. *Fertil. Steril* 65:377–381.

14. Randall J.M. and Templeton A. 1991. Transvaginal sonographic assessment of follicular and sonographic growth in spontaneous and clomiphene citrate cycles. *Fert Steril* 67:256–260.

14

Factors Influencing IUI Outcome: Timing and Number of Inseminations per Cycle

Astrid E.P. Cantineau and Ben Cohlen

Introduction

Timing of insemination is probably one of the most important factors influencing treatment outcome. Various methods have been described for timing intra-uterine insemination (IUI) depending on, among other things, the use of ovarian hyperstimulation, the availability of ultrasound and laboratory facilities to determine luteinizing hormone (LH) levels within a reasonable time frame and of course, expenses. What is the perfect moment to perform the insemination? And when we cannot determine this moment accurately, is it cost-effective to repeat the procedure after 12 or 24 hours to increase the chances of pregnancy? Most of the national and international guidelines advise a single IUI per cycle. However, double insemination may be the answer when more dominant follicles, which rupture with different time-intervals, are available due to ovarian hyperstimulation. Evidence on optimal timing and frequency of IUI will be discussed in this chapter.

Optimal Timing of Insemination

Since oocytes and spermatozoa have a limited period of survival, adequate timing of the insemination is essential for the success of IUI. It has been postulated that ideally, the insemination should be performed just before or maximally 10 hours after ovulation.

There are several methods for timing IUI, of which LH testing and monitoring of follicle development by ultrasound combined with human chorionic gonadotrophin (hCG) injection are most often applied. In cycles with ovarian hyperstimulation, hCG is usually given to induce ovulation. When the dominant follicle(s) reach a mean diameter of approximately 18 mm, hCG is applied in a dosage of 5000 IU. A frequently cited but small (37 cycles) prospective study revealed that ovulation occurs between 34 and 46 hours after the hCG injection (LOE 1b).[1] All patients were monitored by ultrasound with 1 hour interval from 32 hours after hCG injection onward until rupture of the first follicle. In 66%, the largest follicle was the first one to rupture. The mean time interval from hCG administration to follicular rupture was 38.3 hours. This suggests that the optimal timing for insemination would be around 38 hours after hCG administration.

The other approach, waiting for a spontaneous LH surge to occur, is more often applied in natural cycles. In natural cycles ovulation takes place from 24 to 56 hours after the onset of the LH rise, with a mean time of 32 hours.

A few randomized studies on optimal timing of IUI compared hCG injection with urinary LH detection in stimulated cycles. Pooling the results showed no significantly higher pregnancy rate with one of the investigated methods (LOE 1a).[2] The dropout rate in the LH groups was high due to failure to detect an LH surge with urinary detection kits (31% of all cycles), which is disappointing for women undergoing this treatment. Costs were not compared as a secondary outcome in this review.

An alternative way is to detect LH in serum to overcome the effect of false negative urinary LH tests. One recent prospective study[3] compared serum LH detection with hCG triggering in natural cycles. The results revealed a significantly higher pregnancy rate (22.7% versus 10.7%) when IUI was performed 36 hours after an LH rise (defined as a rise of 180% above the latest serum value available) compared to IUI 36 hours after 5000 IU hCG, applied when a dominant follicle reached the size of 17 mm or more. The high pregnancy rate observed is explained by the fact that a large number of included patients were not subfertile. The explanation for the difference in results between both groups might be related to specific LH-induced changes in the endometrium that favor embryo implantation. Furthermore, if hCG is triggered prematurely, the oocyte will be immature and pregnancy will not occur, resulting in a lower pregnancy rate than expected. In conclusion, the use of LH for timing ovulation in natural cycles might be the preferred strategy, although it is questionable whether the results can be extrapolated to a subfertile population. Finally, this strategy might be cost-effective when pregnancy rates double although it might result in more clinic visits and blood withdrawals leading to increased costs per cycle.

Less frequently used timing modalities are (1) injection of a GnRH agonist or (2) recombinant human LH for final oocyte maturation and triggering ovulation, (3) timing with ultrasound alone, and (4) timing based on basal body temperature (BBT) charts. Regarding the use of a GnRH agonist for induction of ovulation and timing IUI, three randomized controlled studies compared the agonist with hCG injection. The pooled effect reported no significant difference between both treatment modalities (LOE 1a).[2] For the other methods of timing IUI mentioned above, prospective trials with adequate trial design are lacking.

It can be concluded that none of the evidence showed that one of the available timing methods is superior to another. Patient's convenience and costs should therefore be involved in decision making.

Not only the method of timing but also the time interval between induction of ovulation and the actual insemination is of paramount importance. Two randomized controlled studies compared different time intervals, namely 32 to 34 hours versus 38 to 40 hours after hCG[4] and 24 hours versus 36 hours after hCG administration.[5] The former included 75 couples and reported no significant difference in pregnancy rates per cycle. The latter included 204 couples and reported a pregnancy rate per cycle of 15% when the insemination was performed 36 hours after hCG injection versus 8.7% when the insemination was performed 24 hours after hCG. However, this difference was not statistically significant (LOE Ib). Finally, one study included in the meta-analysis on the effect of double insemination compared single IUI with two different timing protocols of double IUI. Significantly more pregnancies were reported when IUI was performed 12 and 34 hours after hCG compared to the group where IUI was performed 34 and 60 hours after hCG.

In short, it can be concluded that the available up-to-date evidence suggests that a more flexible approach in timing IUI after hCG is possible, but the proverb of "rather too soon than too late" should be applied here.

Number of Inseminations per Cycle

To bypass the difficulty of optimal timing of IUI, a second insemination in the same cycle can be performed. Increasing the number of inseminations per cycle from one to two may increase the probability of conception. However, there has been no consensus in the literature to date and compared with single IUI, a second IUI adds to the treatment costs and psychological burden. Various randomized controlled trials and systematic reviews have been published on this subject since the early nineties of the previous century, both with different conclusions.

Recently, a systematic review based on six randomized controlled trials (>800 couples) concluded that double IUI does not result in higher pregnancy rates compared with single IUI treatment in women with unexplained subfertility undergoing ovarian hyperstimulation (LOE 1a).[6] On the contrary, a systematic *Cochrane Review*, based on more than 1,750 couples, concluded that double insemination resulted in a statistically significant higher pregnancy rate per couple (LOE 1a).[7] The main difference between these two reviews is that the former included couples with unexplained subfertility only. The latter review assessed the effect of double IUI in women with different causes of subfertility, such as unexplained male subfertility and endometriosis. This causes clinical heterogeneity, which should be taken into account when interpreting the results. One large study included in the meta-analysis reported a significantly higher pregnancy rate with double IUI only in couples suffering from mild male factor subfertility. A good explanation why significantly more pregnancies (up to 20% per cycle) were seen in the male subfertility group was lacking. Thus, we can conclude that for unexplained subfertility a single IUI is sufficient while in case of a male factor the discussion seems ongoing.

Searching for new evidence resulted in three recently published randomized controlled trials with adequate concealment of allocation comparing single versus double IUI.[8–10] The former two studies included couples with unexplained subfertility only and reported no significant difference between single or double IUI in line with the review of Polyzos and coworkers. The latter study[10] included subfertile couples diagnosed with mild male or unexplained factor. Their analysis did not report higher pregnancy rates for double (7.7%) compared to single IUI (10.4%) in the male subfertility group. Incorporating this new evidence in the existing meta-analysis did not change the direction of the effect; double IUI still resulted in significantly more pregnancies per couple (OR 1.5, 95% CI 1.2 to 1.9) when including all types of subfertility. Ideally, a meta-analysis of individual patient data should be performed.

Another hypothesis postulated was that cycles with multi-follicular development would benefit from double insemination only. The studies that reported a significant effect of double IUI stated a mean of three dominant follicles compared to a mean of 1.7 dominant follicles in studies, which did not report a significant difference between single or double IUI. A prospective study that randomized between single and double insemination taking into account the number of follicles could not find any difference in live birth rates between single and double IUI in ovarian hyperstimulation cycles with multi-follicular development (LOE 1b).[10]

In conclusion, double IUI should only be advised when proven effective, since a second IUI adds to the costs and psychological burden, which should be taken into account in decision making. For male factor subfertility this remains to be defined.

Conclusions

The perfect moment to perform IUI has always been defined around the moment of ovulation 38 hours after hCG injection. The current available evidence suggests a wider time frame in which the insemination can be performed from 12 to 36 hours after hCG injection. Most guidelines advised a single well-timed IUI until now. Repeating the insemination procedure in the same cycle is not effective in couples suffering from unexplained subfertility. For male subfertility one study only reported a positive effect of double insemination. The reported results of this latter study should be confirmed in other randomized controlled trials in the future (see also Tables 14.1 and 14.2).

TABLE 14.1

Statements of Chapter 14

Statement	Level of Evidence (LOE)
With regard to pregnancy rates there is no significant difference between timing IUI with hCG injection or urinary LH surge detection	1a
In natural cycles, timing of IUI with LH surge detection in serum revealed a significantly higher pregnancy rate compared to timing with hCG triggering	1b
The optimal time interval between hCG injection and IUI seems to be between 12 and 36 hours	1b
Double IUI does not result in higher pregnancy rates compared with single IUI treatment in women with unexplained subfertility undergoing ovarian hyperstimulation	1a
Double IUI results in higher pregnancy rates compared with single IUI in couples with male factor subfertility	1a
In cycles with multi-follicular development, double IUI does not enhance live birth rates significantly compared with single IUI	1b

TABLE 14.2

Recommendations of Chapter 14

Recommendation	Grade Strength
Timing of IUI can be performed with LH surge detection or hCG injection	A
Timing of IUI should be performed between 12 to 36 hours after hCG injection	A
In couples with unexplained subfertility, one adequately timed IUI is sufficient	A
In couples with mild male subfertility, double IUI should be performed in research setting	A
The frequency of insemination should not depend on multi-follicular growth	A

REFERENCES

1. Andersen A.G., Als-Nielsen B., Hornnes P.J., and Franch Andersen L. 1995. Time interval from human chorionic gonadotrophin (HCG) injection to follicular rupture. *Hum Reprod* 10(12):3202–5.
2. Cantineau A.E.P., Janssen M.J., and Cohlen B.J. 2010. Synchronized approach for intrauterine insemination in subfertile couples. *Cochrane Database of Systematic Reviews* 4.
3. Kyrou D., Kolibianakis E.M., Fatemi H.M., Grimbizis G.F., Theodoridis T.D., Camus M., Tournaye H., Tarlatzis B.C., and Devroey P. 2012. Spontaneous triggering of ovulation versus HCG administration in patients undergoing IUI: A prospective randomized study. *Reprod Biomed Online* 25:278–83.
4. Claman P., Wilkie V., and Collins D. 2004. Timing intrauterine insemination either 33 or 39 hours after administration of human chorionic gonadotrophin yields the same pregnancy rates as after superovulation therapy. *Fertil Steril* 82(1):13–6.
5. Rahman S.M., Karmakar D., Malhotra N., and Kumar S. 2011. Timing of intrauterine insemination: An attempt to unravel the enigma. *Arch Gynecol Obstet* 284(4):1023–7.
6. Polyzos N.P., Tzioras S., Mauri D., and Tatsioni A. 2010. Double versus single intrauterine insemination for unexplained infertility: A meta-analysis of randomized trials. *Fertil Steril* 94(4):1261–6.
7. Cantineau A.E.P., Heineman M.J., and Cohlen B.J. 2009. Single versus double intrauterine insemination in stimulated cycles for subfertile couples. *Cochrane Database of Systematic Reviews* 2.
8. Malhotra N., Gupta S., Rehman S.M., Roy K.K., Kumar S., and Agarwal A. 2007. Comparison of single vs. double intrauterine insemination in unexplained infertility—A randomized control trial. *Fertil Steril* 88:S102.
9. Rahman S.M., Malhotra N., Kumar S., Roy K.K., and Agarwal A. 2010. A randomized controlled trial comparing the effectiveness of single versus double intrauterine insemination in unexplained infertility. *Fertil Steril* 94(7):2913–5.
10. Bagis T., Haydardedeoglu B., Kilicdag E.B., Cok T., Simsek E., and Parlakgumus A.H. 2010. Single versus double intrauterine insemination in multi-follicular ovarian hyperstimulation cycles: A randomized trial. *Hum Reprod* 25(7):1684–90.

15

Factors Influencing IUI Outcome: Site of Insemination in Therapeutic Donor Insemination

Femke P.A.L. Kop and Monique H. Mochtar

Introduction

Therapeutic donor insemination (TDI) is performed in case of severe male subfertility, to prevent vertical transmission of a genetic defect, and to achieve pregnancy in lesbian couples and single women. To prevent transmission of sexually transmitted diseases such as human immunodeficiency virus (HIV) and hepatitis B, TDI is performed with cryopreserved donor sperm,[1] even though pregnancy rates per cycle are lower for cryopreserved sperm than for fresh sperm.[2]

Methods

There are two techniques for insemination for TDI: through the intra-uterine insemination (IUI) or the intracervical (ICI) route. It is currently unknown which of the two insemination techniques is most effective, in terms of ongoing pregnancy rate.

Results

A recent *Cochrane Review*, totaling three randomized controlled trials and one crossover trial (207 patients), suggests a higher ongoing pregnancy rate for IUI with ovarian stimulation (OH) compared to ICI/OH in the first six cycles (OR 1.98, 95% CI 1.85–3.73). Multiple pregnancy rates, which are often the result of OH, did not differ between both techniques (OR 2.19, 95% CI 0.79–6.07)[3] but both IUI/OH and ICI/OH were associated with relatively high multiple pregnancy rates, 14.4 and 6.7%, respectively. IUI/OH is a well-known treatment for couples diagnosed with unexplained subfertility. Comparable high multiple pregnancy rates are described in subfertile couples.[4] In subfertile women the rationale of applying OH is to increase the number of oocytes per cycle to improve pregnancy rates, but the number of growing follicles can only be controlled to a limited extent. Therefore, multiple pregnancies are an inherent risk of this treatment strategy.[5] Because women applying for TDI are not subfertile, the addition of OH for these women is even more controversial and data on unstimulated insemination techniques are therefore important (see also Tables 15.1 and 15.2).

Discussion

The evidence on the effectiveness of IUI and ICI without ovarian stimulation is however very limited. Only six small randomized crossover trials, conducted between 1990 and 2001, entailing 348 women, have investigated the benefit of IUI compared to ICI. One study was published as an abstract only, data on the

TABLE 15.1

Statements of Chapter 15

Statement	Level of Evidence (LOE)
IUI/OH increases ongoing pregnancy rates compared to ICI/OH in TDI	1a
ICI by using a cervical cap increases pregnancy rates compared to standard ICI by straw	1b
Adding OH to inseminations for TDI results in high multiple pregnancy rates	3

TABLE 15.2

Recommendations of Chapter 15

Recommendation	Grade Strength
Women applying for TDI are not subfertile, while adding OH in TDI results in higher multiple pregnancy rates, we therefore recommend to start IUI or ICI in unstimulated cycles	C

number of patients and treatment cycles were not available. A pregnancy rate of 7 and 4.2% was mentioned, however, it is not clear if these pregnancy rates were per cycle or per patient.[6] The data of the remaining five studies were pooled to a total of 500 cycles of IUI and 490 cycles of ICI in 348 women. A clinical pregnancy rate of 14% for IUI per cycle and 6.3% for ICI per cycle (OR 2.3, 95% CI 1.5–3.6) was found.[7–11] Moreover, data on the method of randomization and pre-crossover data were not available, which makes it hard to interpret these data. Furthermore, data on multiple pregnancy rates were also not available.[6–11]

It is noteworthy to mention that in all studies ICI was performed without using a cervical cap with an intracervical reservoir. Using a straw instead of a cervical cap in ICI leads to significantly lower pregnancy rates (5.9% compared to 15% per cycle) (OR 0.4, 95% CI 0.2–0.7).[12]

In conclusion, it is unknown which insemination technique, IUI or ICI, is most effective in terms of ongoing pregnancy rate. Since women applying for TDI are not subfertile and multiple pregnancy rates are high for both IUI/OH and ICI/OH, an insemination technique without OH is recommended. What needs to be studied is the (cost-) effectiveness of IUI compared to ICI, with a cervical cap in unstimulated cycles in terms of ongoing pregnancy rate. This should be the subject of future research.

REFERENCES

1. British Andrology Society. 1999. British Andrology Society guidelines for the screening of semen donors for donor insemination. *Human Reproduction* 14(7):1823–6.
2. Subak L.L., Adamson D., and Boltz N.L. 1992. Therapeutic donor insemination: A prospective randomized trial of fresh versus frozen sperm. *American Journal of Obstetrics & Gynecology* June:1597–604.
3. Besselink D.E., Farquhar C., Kremer J.A.M., Majoribanks J. et al. 2009. Cervical insemination versus intrauterine insemination of donor sperm for subfertility. *Cochrane.* doi: 10.1002/14651858.CD000317.pub3.
4. Steures P., Van der Steeg J.W., Hompes P.G.A., Van der Veen F. et al. 2007. Intrauterine insemination in The Netherlands. *Reprod Biomed Online* 14:110–6.
5. Fauser B.C., Devroey P., and Macklon N.S. 2005. Multiple birth resulting from ovarian stimulation for subfertility treatment. *Lancet* 365:1807–16. doi: 10.1016/S0140-6736(05)66478-1.
6. Alexander C., Lafferty A., Smith C., McNally W. et al. 1994. Treatment of male infertility: A comparison of DI and IUID. Abstracts of 2nd International Meeting of the BFS. Glasgow.
7. Byrd W., Bradshaw K., Carr B., Edman C. et al. 1990. A prospective randomized study of pregnancy rates following intrauterine and intracervical insemination using frozen donor sperm. *Fertility & Sterility* 53:521–7.
8. Peters A., Hecht B., Wentz A, and Jeyendran R. 1993. Comparison of the methods of artificial insemination on the incidence of conception in single unmarried women. *Fertility & Sterility* 59:121–4.
9. Pistorius L.R., Kruger T.F., De Villier A., and Van der Merwe J.P. 1993. A comparative study using prepared and unprepared frozen semen for donor insemination. *Archives of Andrology* 36:81–6.
10. Williams D., Moley K., Cholewa C., Odem R. et al. 1995. Does intrauterine insemination offer an advantage to cervical cap insemination in a donor insemination program? *Fertility & Sterility* 63:295–8.

11. Carroll N. and Palmer J.R. 2001. A comparison of intrauterine versus intracervical insemination in fertile single women. *Fertility & Sterility* 75:656–60.
12. Flierman P.A., Hogerzeil H.V., and Hemrika D.J. 1997. A prospective, randomized, cross-over comparison of two methods of artificial insemination by donor on the incidence of conception: Intracervical insemination by straw versus cervical cap. *Human Reproduction* 12:1945–8.

16

Factors Influencing IUI Outcome: Immobilization after IUI

Inge M. Custers

Since the early 1950s several studies have investigated sperm migration and survival in the female genital tract. Spermatozoa were found to reach the site of fertilization—the fallopian tubes—as soon as two to ten minutes after intracervical insemination.[2–5,7] Considering these studies, one might expect that results after intra-uterine insemination (IUI) are regardless of the female position directly after insemination. However, two randomized studies, one mono-center (n = 116 couples) and one multi-center randomized controlled trial (n = 391 couples) concluded otherwise. It was found that patients who receive IUI for male factor-, cervical factor-, or unexplained subfertility had a significantly higher cumulative ongoing pregnancy rate and live birth rate after three cycles if randomized for a short period of immobilization (10 to 15 minutes) subsequent to insemination compared to immediate mobilization. In the mono-center trial, a cumulative pregnancy rate per couple of 29% in the group that remained in supine position was found versus 10% in the immediate mobilization group (Relative Risk [RR] not mentioned in the article).[6] In the multi-center trial a cumulative ongoing pregnancy rate per couple of 27% versus 18% was found in favor of immobilization (RR 1.50; 95% CI 1.1–2.2; for a live birth RR 1.60; 95% CI 1.1–2.4).[1] Time to pregnancy was also significantly shorter in the group of patients that remained immobilized for a short period of time. In both studies women remained in the same chair as where the insemination was performed, no further adjustments to the female position were made.[1,6]

Although data on a possible dose effect is lacking, it is not likely pregnancy rates continue to rise after prolongation of immobilization after 15 minutes. A possible explanation might be that after immediate mobilization leakage of processed semen from the cervix and vagina occurs or expulsion of semen through uterine contractions and subsequent loss from the vagina.

In conclusion, immobilization for 10 to 15 minutes after artificial homologous IUI significantly increases cumulative ongoing pregnancy rates and live birth rates and shortens time to pregnancy.

TABLE 16.1

Statements of Chapter 16

Statement	Level of Evidence (LOE)
Spermatozoa reach the fallopian tube as soon as 2 minutes after insemination[2–5,7]	2b
10 to 15 minutes immobilization subsequent to IUI, with or without ovarian stimulation, significantly improves cumulative ongoing pregnancy rates and live birth rates[1,6]	1b

TABLE 16.2

Recommendations of Chapter 16

Recommendation	Grade Strength
At least 10 to 15 minutes of immobilization should be applied after every IUI	A

REFERENCES

1. Custers I.M., Flierman P.A., Maas P., Cox T. et al. 2009. Immobilisation versus immediate mobilisation after intrauterine insemination: Randomised controlled trial. *BMJ* 339:b4080. doi: 10.1136/bmj.b4080.
2. Hafez W.E. 1979. *In vivo* and *in vitro* sperm penetration in cervical mucus. *Acta Eur Fertil* 10(2):41–49.
3. Kissler S., Siebzehnruebl E., Kohl J., Mueller A. et al. 2004. Uterine contractility and directed sperm transport assessed by hysterosalpingoscintigraphy (HSSG) and intrauterine pressure (IUP) measurement. *Acta obstet Gynaecol Scand* 83:369–374.
4. Kunz G., Beil D., Deininger H., Wildt L. et al. 1996. The dynamics of rapid sperm transport through the female genital tract: Evidence from vaginal sonography of uterine persitalsis and hysterosalpingoscintigraphy. *Hum Reprod* 11:627–632.
5. Rubenstein, B.B., Strauss H., Lazarus M.L., and Hankin H. 1951. Sperm survival in women. *Fertil Steril* 2:15–19.
6. Saleh A., Tan S.L., Biljan M.M., and Tulandi T. 2000. A randomized study of the effect of 10 minutes of bedrest after intrauterine insemination. *Fertil Steril* 74:509–511.
7. Settlage D.S., Motoshima M., and Tredway D.R. 1973. Sperm transport from the externa cervical os to the fallopian tubes in women: A time and quantitation study. *Fertil Steril* 24:655–661.

17

Factors Influencing IUI Outcome: Ovarian Hyperstimulation

Ben Cohlen, Rosa Tur, and Rosario Buxaderas

Introduction

The rationale behind intra-uterine insemination (IUI) is increasing the number of available motile spermatozoa at the site of fertilization. In addition to increasing the number of spermatozoa, one can also increase the number of available oocytes by applying ovarian hyperstimulation. With the use of hyperstimulation one might also overcome subtle cycle disturbances, and increase the accuracy of timing of the insemination. On the other hand, applying hyperstimulation increases the probability of achieving multiple pregnancies. Therefore, ovarian hyperstimulation in IUI programs should be applied when proven effective only. One should make a distinction between ovarian hyperstimulation (striving after multi-follicular development) and ovulation induction for women with anovulation (striving after mono-follicular development and ovulation). This chapter will focus on the indications for IUI in combination with (mild) ovarian hyperstimulation, its methods, and risks.

Overview of Existing Evidence

As stated in Chapter 4, IUI in combination with (mild) ovarian hyperstimulation has been proven effective in couples with unexplained subfertility (LOE 1a), with minimal to mild endometriosis (LOE 1b), and mild male subfertility defined as an average total motile sperm count above 10 million (LOE 1b). In couples with a cervical factor or moderate male subfertility the addition of ovarian hyperstimulation has been proven ineffective (LOE 1b and 1a).

The goal of ovarian hyperstimulation should be the development of two to three dominant follicles (LOE 1a).[1] This strategy, however, increases the risk of achieving a multiple pregnancy. The line drawn between maximizing the probability of conception and the unacceptable high percentages of multiple pregnancy rates is thin.

Several drugs are available to achieve ovarian hyperstimulation. Probably the oldest one is clomiphene citrate (CC) in dosages of 50–150 mg per day for 5 days starting early in the cycle. Being an oral drug and relatively cheap, it is a popular option, easy to apply, although side effects, such as hot flushes and headaches are present. Being an anti-estrogen, one should be aware of its negative action on the endometrium. This might explain the observed lower pregnancy rates with CC compared with other drugs.[2] Furthermore, the use of CC for ovarian hyperstimulation does not prevent the occurrence of multiple pregnancies.[3] Tamoxifen might also be chosen instead of CC. Although tamoxifen might have a less negative effect on the endometrium, compared with CC, it does not seem to further improve pregnancy rates significantly (LOE 1b).

In addition to CC, gonadotrophins are applied frequently. These drugs are more expensive, invasive, and potent compared with CC. A meta-analysis clearly shows gonadotrophins to be more effective compared with CC (Figure 17.1) (LOE 1a).[3] Different types of gonadotrophins are available but a meta-analysis of

Pregnancy rate per couple

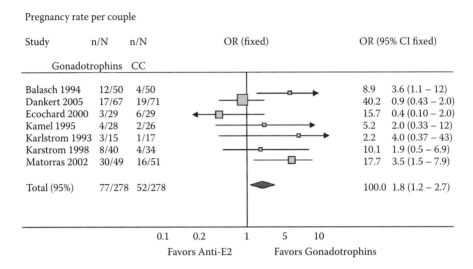

Study	n/N	n/N		OR (95% CI fixed)
	Gonadotrophins	CC		
Balasch 1994	12/50	4/50	8.9	3.6 (1.1 – 12)
Dankert 2005	17/67	19/71	40.2	0.9 (0.43 – 2.0)
Ecochard 2000	3/29	6/29	15.7	0.4 (0.10 – 2.0)
Kamel 1995	4/28	2/26	5.2	2.0 (0.33 – 12)
Karlstrom 1993	3/15	1/17	2.2	4.0 (0.37 – 43)
Karstrom 1998	8/40	4/34	10.1	1.9 (0.5 – 6.9)
Matorras 2002	30/49	16/51	17.7	3.5 (1.5 – 7.9)
Total (95%)	77/278	52/278	100.0	1.8 (1.2 – 2.7)

0.1   0.2   1   5   10

Favors Anti-E2   Favors Gonadotrophins

FIGURE 17.1 Ovarian hyperstimulation with gonadotrophins compared with ovarian hyperstimulation with clomiphene citrate.

trials comparing urinary with recombinant gonadotrophins did not show one type to be superior to the other (LOE 1a).[3] Furthermore, there is an ongoing discussion regarding the optimal dose. Doubling the daily dose of gonadotrophins from 75 IU to 150 IU does not result in improvement of treatment outcome while it significantly increases the chances of achieving a multiple pregnancy (LOE 1a).[3] When a very low-dose regimen is given on alternating days extremely low pregnancy rates are seen, which makes it plausible that a minimum acquired dose of gonadotrophins is needed.

More recently, aromatase inhibitors are used for ovarian hyperstimulation in IUI programs. The rationale is that aromatase inhibitors do not have a negative effect on the endometrium and cervical mucus known from CC. However, compared with CC, these drugs do not seem to improve treatment outcome significantly while being more expensive (LOE 1a).[3] Thus, there seems to be little place for aromatase inhibitors in IUI programs.

It has been shown that in stimulated IUI cycles, spontaneous LH surges occur frequently, up to one-third of all cycles, and when not monitored, timing of the insemination might be influenced negatively (i.e., too late), resulting in significantly lower pregnancy rates (LOE 2).[4] To prevent spontaneous LH surges, GnRH agonists and antagonists can be applied in IUI programs. The use of GnRH agonists might result in more aggressive stimulation protocols, thus resulting in higher multiple pregnancy rates.[2] In addition to this disadvantage, evidence reveals that until now there seems no benefit of GnRH-agonists while they significantly increase the costs per treatment cycle (LOE 1a).[2] GnRH antagonists are also used in IUI programs to suppress spontaneous LH surges. They are often applied after a fixed number of days of stimulation. They do not have the disadvantages of agonists with regard to more aggressive stimulation protocols. Recently however, it has been shown that GnRH antagonists that seemed promising in the beginning, are not cost-effective in IUI programs (Figure 17.2) (LOE 1a).[5] One might still apply GnRH antagonists in couples with previous undetected spontaneous LH surges or to avoid insemination in the weekends (although large fertility centers should be able to inseminate at least 6 days a week). An alternative has been suggested by Al-Inany et al. by applying CC after hMG stimulation to suppress LH surges (LOE 1b).[6] Although LH surges were suppressed successfully this treatment option did not increase pregnancy rates.

Recently, several small randomized trials found a significant benefit of the use of luteal support with vaginally applied progesterone in stimulated IUI cycles (LOE 1b). Before this drug is introduced in IUI programs on a large scale, a multi-center placebo-controlled double-blinded trial with cost-effectiveness analyses seems mandatory to confirm these first promising results.

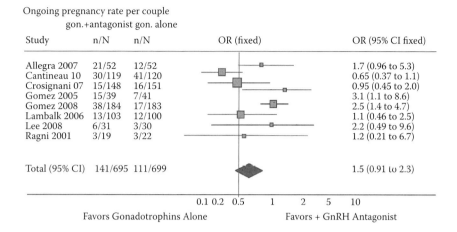

Ongoing pregnancy rate per couple

Study	gon.+antagonist n/N	gon. alone n/N	OR (fixed)	OR (95% CI fixed)
Allegra 2007	21/52	12/52		1.7 (0.96 to 5.3)
Cantineau 10	30/119	41/120		0.65 (0.37 to 1.1)
Crosignani 07	15/148	16/151		0.95 (0.45 to 2.0)
Gomez 2005	15/39	7/41		3.1 (1.1 to 8.6)
Gomez 2008	38/184	17/183		2.5 (1.4 to 4.7)
Lambalk 2006	13/103	12/100		1.1 (0.46 to 2.5)
Lee 2008	6/31	3/30		2.2 (0.49 to 9.6)
Ragni 2001	3/19	3/22		1.2 (0.21 to 6.7)
Total (95% CI)	141/695	111/699		1.5 (0.91 to 2.3)

Favors Gonadotrophins Alone   Favors + GnRH Antagonist

FIGURE 17.2 Ovarian hyperstimulation with GnRH antagonist compared with ovarian hyperstimulation without GnRH antagonist.

It is clear that when ovarian hyperstimulation is applied multiple pregnancies will occur. Both studies in The Netherlands as the ESHRE registry of treatment outcome show that the probability of achieving a twin pregnancy is approximately 10% while triplets occur in less than 1% of the pregnancies (LOE 3). Mild ovarian hyperstimulation with 50 to 75 IU FSH per day in combination with strict cancellation criteria should minimize these risks. The occurrence and prevention of multiple pregnancies is discussed in Chapters 26 and 27.

Discussion

As stated before, the line drawn between increasing pregnancy rates with ovarian hyperstimulation (OH) and achieving multiple pregnancies is thin. Therefore, OH should only be applied when proven effective and safe. Until now, there seems to be a place for OH in combination with IUI in couples with unexplained subfertility, mild male subfertility almost resembling couples with unexplained subfertility, and couples with minimal to mild endometriosis. Ovarian hyperstimulation should be mild and gonadotrophins seem to be the most effective drug in dosages of 50–75 IU per day. When mono-follicular development is achieved the dosage can be increased safely during the next treatment cycle with 25–37.5 IU per day. Strict ultrasound monitoring of each stimulated cycle is mandatory. One should strive after two dominant follicles larger than 16 mm but all follicles larger than 10 mm should be measured and taken into account when defining cancellation criteria. When resources are scarce, CC (100 mg per day for 5 days) can be applied although CC seems less effective and might have a negative effect on the endometrium. There seems to be no place for aromatase inhibitors, GnRH agonist, or antagonists in OH/IUI programs. One should be aware of spontaneous LH surges and apply hCG ovulation induction not too late. Whether one should measure LH daily to anticipate these surges has not been proven cost-effective so far.

The evidence until now that support the use of OH in IUI programs is largely derived from studies applying aggressive stimulation protocols with 150 IU FSH per day. Therefore, future trials should focus on the cost-effectiveness of mild ovarian hyperstimulation only. Furthermore, prediction models should be constructed that support clinicians in applying the appropriate dosage of daily FSH to achieve two follicles. New tools like antral follicle count, antimullerian hormone, but also factors as age, BMI, and smoking might be predictors of ovarian response. Finally, because OH/IUI results in significantly lower pregnancy rates compared with IVF, OH/IUI should not be applied extensively and future research should focus on identifying those couples that benefit from OH/IUI and those that do not (see also Tables 17.1 and 17.2).

TABLE 17.1

Statements of Chapter 17

Statement	Level of Evidence (LOE)
IUI in combination with (mild) ovarian hyperstimulation has been proven effective in couples with unexplained subfertility	1a
IUI in combination with (mild) ovarian hyperstimulation seems effective in couples with minimal to mild endometriosis	1b
IUI in combination with (mild) ovarian hyperstimulation seems effective in couples with mild male subfertility defined as an average total motile sperm count above 10 million	1b
The goal of ovarian hyperstimulation should be the development of two to three dominant follicles	1a
Gonadotrophins used for ovarian hyperstimulation in IUI programs are more effective compared to clomiphene citrate	1a
Doubling the daily dose of gonadotrophins from 75 IU to 150 IU does not result in improvement of treatment outcome while it significantly increases the chances of achieving a multiple pregnancy	1a
Aromatase inhibitors used for ovarian hyperstimulation are, compared with CC, not more effective while being more expensive	1a
Spontaneous LH surges occur frequently in stimulated IUI cycles and might result in lower pregnancy rates	2
Both GNRH agonists and antagonists are not (cost-) effective in ovarian stimulation/IUI programs	1a
The use of luteal support with vaginally applied progesterone in stimulated IUI cycles might increase pregnancy rates but more randomized trials are warranted	1b
The probability of achieving a twin pregnancy in stimulated IUI cycles is approximately 10% while triplets occur in less than 1% of the pregnancies	3

TABLE 17.2

Recommendations of Chapter 17

Recommendation	Grade Strength
Mild ovarian hyperstimulation in combination with IUI should be applied in couples with unexplained or mild male subfertility and in couples with minimal to mild endometriosis	A
When ovarian hyperstimulation is applied one should strive after the occurrence of two follicles (using mild stimulation starting with 50–75 IU FSH per day) and gonadotrophins are the drugs of first choice	A
Aromatase inhibitors, GNRH agonists, or GNRH antagonists should not be used in IUI programs	A
Luteal support in ovarian hyperstimulation/IUI programs should be applied in randomized trials only	B

REFERENCES

1. Van Rumste M.M., Custers I.M., Van der Veen F., Van Wely M., Evers J.L., and Mol B.W. 2008. The influence of the number of follicles on pregnancy rates in intrauterine insemination with ovarian stimulation: A meta-analysis. *Hum Reprod Update* November 14(6):563–70.
2. Biljan M.M., Mahutte N.G., Tulandi T., and Tan S.L. 1999. Prospective randomized double-blind trial of the correlation between time of administration and antiestrogenic effects of clomiphene citrate on reproductive end organs. *Fertil Steril* April 71(4):633–8.
3. Cantineau A.E., Cohlen B.J., and Heineman M.J. 2007. Ovarian stimulation protocols (anti-oestrogens, gonadotrophins with and without GnRH agonists/antagonists) for intrauterine insemination (IUI) in women with subfertility. *Cochrane Database Syst Rev* (2):CD005356.
4. Cantineau A.E. and Cohlen B.J. 2007. The prevalence and influence of luteinizing hormone surges in stimulated cycles combined with intrauterine insemination during a prospective cohort study. *Fertil Steril* July 88(1):107–12.

5. Cantineau A.E., Cohlen B.J., Klip H., and Heineman M.J. 2011. The addition of GnRH antagonists in intrauterine insemination cycles with mild ovarian hyperstimulation does not increase live birth rates—A randomized, double-blinded, placebo-controlled trial. *Hum Reprod* May 26(5):1104–11.
6. Al-Inany H., Azab H., El-Khayat W., Nada A., El-Khattan E., and Abou-Setta A.M. 2010. The effectiveness of clomiphene citratein LH surge suppression in women undergoing IUI: A randomized controlled trial. *Fertil Steril* November 94(6):2167–71.

18

Factors Influencing IUI Outcome: Luteal Phase Support

Ahmet Erdem

Intra-uterine insemination (IUI) combined with ovarian hyperstimulation using clomiphene citrate (CC) or gonadotrophin is a commonly used technique for the baseline treatment of couples with mild male factor and unexplained subfertility. Despite its popularity, the effectiveness of the method is still debated as the success rates for IUI cycles widely differ in the literature.

Several factors influence the effectiveness of IUI. These factors may be related to the infertile couples (i.e., age of the female partner, semen parameters, and endometriosis), insemination techniques (i.e., timing and number of IUI, method of sperm preparation) or ovarian hyperstimulation protocols (CC, gonadotophins, gonadotrophin releasing hormone (GnRH) antagonists, luteal phase support). The effects of these factors have been assessed in many studies. However, there are few evidence-based data from prospective randomized studies evaluating the effect of these factors on IUI prognosis. Luteal phase support of the stimulated IUI cycles is one of these factors. For many years, the use of human chorionic gonadotrophin (hCG)/progesterone has become an established clinical practice despite any scientific evidence of benefit. Recently, several prospective randomized studies were published investigating the efficacy of the luteal phase support in IUI cycles with ovarian hyperstimulation. The results obtained from these studies are reviewed in this chapter using evidence-based guidelines.

Ovarian Hyperstimulation and Luteal Phase Function

Luteal phase is the important period of the menstrual cycle in which embryonic implantation occurs. A good quality luteal phase is characterized with adequate progesterone secretion by the corpus luteum and endometrial secretory transformation. Optimum follicular development followed by adequate luteinizing hormone (LH) surge for ovulation and persistent LH secretion are required for adequate luteal phase function. Any factors altering the follicular and hormonal dynamics may have a deleterious effect on luteal phase functions. The supraphysiological hormonal environment caused by ovarian hyperstimulation (OH) for multiple follicular development as well as the GnRH agonists and antagonists that are used in conjunction with OH may influence corpus luteum function and endometrial receptivity for implantation.[1,2]

Corpus luteum function is dependent on LH stimulation. In agonist *in vitro* fertilization (IVF) cycles, suppression of endogenous luteal LH levels by the GnRH agonist leads to shortened luteal phase and low progesterone levels. Low early-midluteal LH levels, decreased progesterone production, and short luteal phase length are also observed in GnRH antagonist IVF cycles without luteal support as in agonist cycles. In addition to these observations, clinical data strongly supports the benefit of luteal progesterone support in GnRH agonist/antagonist IVF cycles.[1]

There is also evidence that luteal phase characteristics might be altered in nonagonist/antagonist ovarian hyperstimulation cycles. LH levels are decreased early in the luteal phase in gonadotrophin stimulated cycles, indicating the effect of ovarian hyperstimulation on inducing luteal phase defect by influencing the mechanisms involved in the regulation of LH secretion.[1] It has been suggested that supraphysiological serum sex steroid concentrations might adversely affect LH secretion via negative feedback on the pituitary–hypothalamic axis, which in turn results with premature luteolysis and defective progesterone secretion.[1]

Ovarian hyperstimulation may also influence receptivity of the endometrium for implantataion. Alterations in endometrial development have been demonstrated in most of the ovarian hyperstimulation protocols. CC as well as aromatase inhibitors and selective estrogen receptor modulators have the potential to influence endometrial receptivity by their anti-estrogenic effects.[2] OH with multi-follicular development has significant effects on luteal endometrium. Advancement in the endometrial histology in the late proliferative phase before ovulation, earlier shift into implantation window, and delay and/or asynchrony in the maturation of mid and late-luteal endometria are the morphological changes detected in OH cycles with gonadotrophin stimulation alone or in combination with GnRH agonist or antagonist suppression.[1,2] Altered hormonal environment with high estrogen or progesterone concentrations before and around the time of ovulation with multi-follicular development or altered estrogen/progesterone ratio have been suggested to affect endometrial development and embryonic implantation.[2]

Luteal Support in IUI Cycles

Although the effectiveness of luteal phase support in improving outcome is evident in IVF cycles with GnRH agonists or antagonists, there was no evidence-based data in mildly stimulated IUI cycles until recently. Three recent randomized trials investigated the impact of luteal phase support in IUI programs.[3–5] These studies were different for the study populations, ovarian hyperstimulation agent and the drug used for luteal phase support (Table 18.1). The stimulation protocol used CC in one study, while low-dose recombinant gonadotrophins were used in the other two studies. The study populations were different between the studies and only unexplained subfertile were included in one study, while male factor infertility and other IUI indications (donor sperm) were included in other studies.

The first publication was investigating the efficacy of luteal support using progesterone gel (Crinone®) in IUI cycles stimulated with recombinant gonadotrophins in a homogenous unexplained subfertile population.[3] A total of 427 IUI cycles of 214 patients were analyzed in this parallel design, randomized study. The live birth rates per cycle (39.4% versus 23.8%, p = 0.01) and per patient (35.8 versus 18.1%, p = 0.003) were significantly higher in patients having vaginal progesterone gel for luteal support as compared to controls. Although the patients were mildly stimulated with a low starting gonadotrophin dose of 75 IUI per day, the follicular response was multi-follicular. The mean serum estradiol levels on the day of hCG injection for ovulation trigger was not compared in the study; however, a severalfold increase in serum sex steroid levels might be expected with a mean of 1.52 dominant follicles and 2.8 intermediate follicles between 9–16 mm diameter per patient on the day of hCG trigger after ovarian hyperstimulation. The luteal phase lengths did not differ between luteal support and control groups (median length of 11.9 versus 12, respectively), but 29% of patients without luteal support had luteal length below median. Interestingly, the clinical abortion rates did not differ between the luteal support and control groups (3.4 versus 3.5, respectively). These findings suggest that luteal support with progesterone improves pregnancy outcome by affecting implantation process in gonadotrophin stimulated IUI cycles.

Recently, the impact of luteal phase support with vaginal progesterone gel (Crinone) in IUI cycles with low-dose recombinant FSH stimulation was assessed in another study.[5] In this prospective study with a relatively small population of heterogeneous infertility etiology (female, male, combined, and unexplained), 71 patients were randomized to supported and unsupported luteal phase in their first cycles. Subsequent cycles were alternated until pregnancy was achieved or a maximum of six cycles. The live birth rate per cycle significantly improved in supported cycles compared to unsupported cycles (35.2% versus 18.9%; p = 0.001). The crossover design is the major negative aspect of this study. Nevertheless, the first cycle analysis revealed similar results. A significantly higher live birth rate was also detected in supported first cycles as compared to unsupported ones (27% versus 8.8%; p = 0.04). Another negative aspect of the study is the heterogeneous study population with regard to the infertility etiology. Sperm parameters may be an important determinant of success in IUI cycles. Thus, the results of the subgroup of couples with male factor should be analyzed separately. The miscarriage rate did not differ between the groups as in the former study.

TABLE 18.3

Characteristics and the Main Results of the Randomized Studies Evaluating the Effect of Luteal Phase Support with Progesterone on the Outcome of Stimulated IUI Cycles

Study	Randomization Method	Concealment of Allocation	Design	Power Calculation	Number of Patients Randomized	Form of Luteal Phase Support	Main Results
Erdem 2008[a]	Computer generated	No	Parallel	No	214	Progesterone 8% vaginal gel (Crinone)	Live birth rate/patient favors luteal support (35.8 versus 18.1%, p = 0.003)
Kyrou 2010[b]	Computer generated	No	Parallel	Yes	468	200 mg/three times daily micronized vaginal progesterone (Utrogestan)	Ongoing pregnancy rate/patient not different between luteal support or no support (8.7% versus 9.3%, p = 0.82)
Maher 2011[c]	Computer generated	No	Crossover	No	71	Progesterone 8% vaginal gel (Crinone)	Live birth rate/cycle favors luteal support (35.2% versus 18.9%; p = 0.001) First cycle live birth rate (27% versus 8.8%; p = 0.04)

[a] Erdem et al., 2009, *Fertil Steril* 91:2508–13.
[b] Kyrou et al., 2010, *Hum Reprod* 25:2501–6.
[c] Maher, 2011, *Eur J Obstet Gynecol Reprod Biol* 157:57–62.

TABLE 18.1

Statements of Chapter 18

Statement	Level of Evidence (LOE)
Luteal phase support using vaginal progesterone improves live birth rates in IUI cycles stimulated with low-dose gonadotrophins in couples with unexplained subfertility	1b
Luteal phase support with vaginal progesterone does not seem to improve pregnancy rates in normo-ovulatory women stimulated with clomiphene citrate for IUI	1b

TABLE 18.2

Recommendations of Chapter 18

Recommendation	Grade Strength
Luteal phase support should be added to IUI cycles mildly stimulated with gonadotrophins in couples with unexplained subfertility	A
Luteal phase support should not be added to clomiphene citrate stimulated IUI cycles of normo-ovulatory women	A

The third study is the only report assessing the effect of luteal support on ongoing pregnancy rates in CC stimulated IUI cycles in normo-ovulatory women.[4] Patients were stimulated with 50 mg per day of CC and were randomized to receive luteal support in the form of vaginal micronized progesterone (Utrogestan® 200 mg) three times a day or to the control group not receiving luteal support. The study population was not homogeneous for IUI indications. Approximately half of the participants had IUI cycles with donor sperm and one fourth of the population had male factor subfertility. The results of the 400 women did not display any significant difference in ongoing pregnancy rates between patients who did or did not receive luteal support (8.7% versus 9.3%, p = 0.82).

Choice of low dose (50 mg) for CC and heterogeneous study population are the shortcomings of the study. Subgroup analyses were absent for male factor and idiopathic subfertile groups. The miscarriage rate did not differ between the groups as in the other two studies. It was concluded that the use of CC for induction did not fulfill the purpose of administration for IUI cycles probably because of its adverse effects on endometrium.

Conclusions

The results of the two randomized controlled trials clearly demonstrate that luteal phase support with progesterone gel increases live birth rates in IUI cycles mildly stimulated with recombinant gonadotrophins in subfertile couples. The results of the one randomized controlled trial did not show any benefit of luteal phase support with vaginal progesterone to improve pregnancy rates in CC stimulated IUI cycles of normo-ovulatory women (see also Tables 18.1 and 18.2).

Although the effectiveness of luteal support in gonadotrophin IUI cycles is well documented in couples with unexplained subfertility, there is yet no data in the subgroup of mild male factor infertility. Further studies are also needed for different progesterone forms and doses, different routes of administration, and the necessity to continue supplementation after pregnancy occurs. Cost-effectiveness of the method is an important issue, which needs to be analyzed in future trials.

REFERENCES

1. Tavanitou A., Albano C., Smitz J., and Devroey P. 2002. Impact of ovarian stimulation on corpus luteum function and embryonic implantation. *J Reprod Immunol* 55(1–2):123–30.
2. Devroey P., Bourgain C., Macklon N.S., and Fauser B.C. 2004. Reproductive biology and IVF: Ovarian stimulation and endometrial receptivity. *Trends Endocrinol Metab* March 15(2):84–90.

3. Erdem A., Erdem M., Atmaca S., and Guler I. 2009. Impact of luteal phase support on pregnancy rates in intrauterine insemination cycles: A prospective randomized study. *Fertil Steril* 91:2508–13.

4. Kyrou D., Fatemi H.M., Tournaye H., and Devroey P. 2010. Luteal phase support in normo-ovulatory women stimulated with clomiphenecitrate for intrauterine insemination: Need or habit? *Hum Reprod* 25:2501–6.

5. Maher M.A. 2011. Luteal phase support may improve pregnancy outcomes during intrauterine insemination cycles. *Eur J Obstet Gynecol Reprod Biol* 157:57–62.

19

Fallopian Sperm Perfusion: Evidence on IUI versus Fallopian Sperm Perfusion

Willem Ombelet, Arne Sunde, and Jarl A. Kahn

Introduction

Conventionally, intra-uterine insemination (IUI) is performed using a relatively small volume of inseminate (~0.3–0.5 ml). Fallopian sperm perfusion (FSP) is a similar procedure using a large volume (4 ml) of inseminate originally described in cases of unexplained infertility and using mild ovarian stimulation with the aim of maturing two follicles.[1] The rationale behind FSP is to create a sperm flushing of the tubes and an overflow of motile spermatozoa closer to the eggs. The final goal is to maximize the chances that gametes will meet and fertilization occurs.[1] In a prospective randomized study, Khan et al.[1] showed that FSP gave higher pregnancy rates compared to conventional IUI in the case of unexplained infertility (OR 4.1, 95% CI 1.2–13.4). In different studies, Kahn et al. showed that FSP maximizes the likelihood that sperm cells were present not only in the uterus, but also in the fallopian tubes and even in the peritoneal space.

Several studies from other research groups have tried to elucidate whether FSP or IUI will give the highest pregnancy rates in the treatment of unexplained infertility. Most of these studies are rather small. Another complicating factor is that in these studies, different stimulation protocols, different utensils, and different catheters have been used. This may well have influenced the outcome of the studies and contributed to the fact that currently there is no clear consensus on whether FSP or IUI is to be advocated in case of nontubal infertility and no severe male factor.

Methods and Materials

According to the inventors, FSP is most successful and only recommended in unexplained infertility cases. According to the first reports the following methods should be followed:

> For FSP the sperm cells are resuspended in 4 ml instead of 0.5 ml culture media. For ovarian stimulation clomiphene citrate 50 mg daily from cycle day 4 to 8 is used in combination with human menopausal gonadotrophins or recombinant FSH 75 IU daily from cycle day 7 to 9. Human chorionic gonadotrophin (hCG) 5000 IU is administered when at least one follicle reaches 17 mm in diameter. The aim is to mature a maximum of two follicles (>15 mm). Cycles with too many maturing follicles (>4) are either canceled or converted to IVF treatment. Insemination is performed 34–36 hours following administration of hCG. The vagina and the cervix are rinsed with sterile saline. For FSP, a 5 ml plastic syringe is filled with 4 ml of the inseminate. A catheter (Frydman embryo transfer catheter, CCD France) with the inseminate is placed into the upper part of the uterine cavity. The insemination is performed rather slowly (~1 ml/minute). An Allis clamp is placed on the cervix to prevent reflux. The Allis clamp is kept in place for some minutes after insemination.

A relationship between the treatment cycle number and pregnancy rate was observed with a clear drop in pregnancy rate after the second treatment cycle. The pregnancy rate in cycles four or more were very low. A maximum of three FSP cycles in case of unexplained infertility is recommended.

Overview of Existing Evidence

In a prospective randomized trial Kahn et al. observed a significantly higher pregnancy rate both per cycle (26.9 versus 9.8%) and per woman treated (46.7 versus 17.9%) for FSP compared to regular IUI in unexplained infertility cases.[1] Several other randomized studies have been done by other clinics with varying results inspiring research groups to do a meta-analysis to decide whether the accumulated data were in favor of FSP or not. Trout and Kemman[2] reported the first meta-analysis and this was followed in 2004 by a *Cochrane Database Structured Review*.[3] Six studies involving 474 couples were included in the meta-analysis. In this Cochrane analysis it was concluded that FSP may be more effective for nontubal subfertility, but the significant heterogeneity should be taken into account. Subgroup analysis suggested that couples with unexplained infertility may benefit from FSP over IUI in terms of higher pregnancy rates (OR 2.88, 95% CI 1.73–4.78). Results suggested the possibility of differential effectiveness of FSP depending on catheter choice.

In 2009 a second Cochrane analysis was performed, including more studies published between 2003 and 2008.[4] Eight studies involving 595 couples were included in this meta-analysis. No difference could be found between FSP and IUI for clinical pregnancy per couple (OR 1.2, 95% CI 0.79 to 1.7). A subgroup analysis, which included couples with unexplained subfertility only (n = 239) did not report any difference between FSP and IUI anymore (OR 1.6, 95% CI 0.89 to 2.8). According to this review FSP does not give higher pregnancy rates that should be compared to classical IUI.[4]

It is of interest that in one of the new studies they used a Foley catheter and obtained much better results with IUI than FSP.[5] It is a concern that Foley catheters seem to be associated with lower pregnancy rates in FSP (3.5). Computing the odds ratio of pregnancies omitting the studies using the Foley catheter give an OR of 2.0 (95% CI 1.3–3.2) in favor of FSP.

Since 2008 only one valuable randomized controlled trial comparing FSP versus IUI in mild-moderate male factor infertility has been published. In this study FSP was more successful than IUI.[7]

Discussion

In the original papers of Kahn et al., FSP turned out to be superior to IUI in unexplained infertility patients. Several variants of FSP have been developed using different forms of catheters, clamps, and devices to perform the insemination itself including different devices for blocking reflux.

Despite the fact that several randomized studies and ensuing meta-analyses presented data suggesting that FSP is more efficient than standard IUI, it is unclear why this method has not replaced the standard IUI protocol. FSP is not more difficult to perform than IUI, it is a well-tolerated technique and side effects or complications are comparable with classical IUI. It might be that the costs of the catheter play a role (see also Tables 19.1 and 19.2).

A complicating factor in the evaluation of FSP is the fact that several and perhaps less efficient variants of FSP have been developed by other research groups. According to two prospective studies, IUI gives better results than FSP if a Foley catheter is used.[6,7] This is in contrast to most other published studies where pregnancy rates obtained with FSP were at least as good as, if not better, than the pregnancy rates obtained with IUI. Whether this observation warrants a clear advice not to use the Foley catheter for FSP is still unclear.[3,5]

Because of the promising results in many studies we believe that a well-powered multi-center prospective randomized trial comparing pregnancy outcome of FSP (without Foley catheter) with regular IUI in case of unexplained and moderate male infertility should be performed. Whether moderate ovarian stimulation has to be added to FSP and regular IUI remains questionable.

TABLE 19.1

Statements of Chapter 19

Statement	Level of Evidence (LOE)
For nontubal subfertility, the results indicate no clear benefit for FSP over IUI	1a
After the exclusion of studies where a Foley catheter was used, FSP resulted in a significantly higher pregnancy rate compared to standard IUI	1a

TABLE 19.2

Recommendations of Chapter 19

Recommendation	Grade Strength
FSP can be used as an alternative treatment option for standard IUI in case of unexplained infertility and no Foley catheter is used	A
In case of unexplained infertility, a maximum of three FSP cycles is recommended	B

REFERENCES

1. Kahn J.A., Sunde A., Koskemies A., von Düring V., Sørdal T., Christensen F., and Molne K. 1993. Fallopian tube sperm perfusion (FSP) versus intra-uterine insemination (IUI) in the treatment of unexplained infertility: A prospective randomized study. *Hum Reprod* 8:890–894.
2. Trout S.W. and Kemman E. 1999. Fallopian sperm perfusion versus intrauterine insemination: A randomized controlled trial and meta-analysis of the literature. *Fertil Steril* 71:881–885.
3. Cantineau A.E.P., Cohlen B.J., Al-Inany H., and Heineman M.J. 2004. Intrauterine insemination versus fallopian tube sperm perfusion for nontubal infertility. *Cochrane Database of Systematic Reviews* (3):CD001502.
4. Cantineau A.E.P., Cohlen B.J., and Heineman M.J. 2009. Intra-uterine insemination versus fallopian tube sperm perfusion for non-tubal infertility. *Cochrane Database Syst Reviews* (2):CD001502.
5. Biacchiardi C.P., Revelli A., Gennarelli G., Rustichelli S., Moffa F., and Massobrio M. 2004. Fallopian tube sperm perfusion versus intrauterine insemination in unexplained infertility: A randomized, prospective, cross-over trial. *Fertil Steril* 81:448–451.
6. Nuojou-Huttunen S., Tuomivaara L., Juntunen K., Tomás C., and Martikainen H. 1997. Comparison of fallopian tube sperm perfusion with intra-uterine insemination in the treatment of infertility. *Fertil Steril* 67:939–942.
7. El-Khayat W., El-Mazny A., Abou-Salem N., Moafy A. 2012. The value of fallopian tube sperm perfusion in the management of mild-moderate male factor infertility. *Int J Gynaecol Obstet* 117(2):178–181.

20

Media Supplements: Platelet Activating Factor Improves Sperm Motility and IUI Outcomes

Linda M. Street, Bonnie Patel, and William E. Roudebush

In many fertility centers, drug-induced ovulation induction followed by intra-uterine insemination (IUI) has become standard therapy for nontubal factor-related infertility. As the initial treatment for infertile couples, IUI is commonly used and seems a cost-effective procedure. The success of IUI depends on many aspects such as the method of ovulation induction as well as seminal parameters. Cumulative pregnancy rates for three cycles have approached those of a single IVF treatment when exogenous gonadotrophins are combined with IUI. Typically, a couple first undergoes a simple IUI cycle without any additives. After this fails, especially in the setting of an abnormal semen analysis, IUI utilizing media supplements may be preferable.

Sperm prior to IUI must be processed first (e.g., density/gradient wash or swim up). This processing of sperm ensures that the most normal motile population is used for conception. For IUI procedures, semen washing is important as it removes prostaglandins, debris, and white blood cells while also reducing the number of nonmotile and morphologically abnormal sperm cells. Additionally, removal of seminal plasma also benefits sperm by enhancing capacitating conditions resulting in the enhancement of sperm motility. A number of sperm motility enhancers have been investigated, including but not limited to: cAMP, human follicular fluid, xanthine, caffeine, pentoxifylline, and platelet-activating factor (PAF). However, since PAF has been primarily used to effectively improve sperm motility and subsequent IUI pregnancy outcomes, this chapter will focus on this naturally occurring and nontoxic substance for use in an IUI program.

Platelet-activating factor (PAF; 1-O-alkyl-2-O-acetyl-sn-glycero-3-phosphorylcholine) is a unique signaling phospholipid that has pleiotropic biologic properties and clearly plays a significant role in reproductive physiology where it influences ovulation, fertilization, preimplantation embryo development, implantation, and parturition. Although the exact mechanisms of PAF action remain unclear, the importance of PAF for normal reproductive function is clear. Exposure of sperm to PAF significantly improves sperm motility,[1] capacitation,[2] and the acrosome reaction.[3]

There is some evidence that the forward progression of sperm is an indicator of potential pregnancy.[4] Forward progression can be measured objectively by rating the sperm according to the following scale: 4 = rapid, 3 = medium, 2 = slow, and 0–1 = static. Once the percent of sperm falling into each of these categories has been determined, to obtain the motility index the percent of sperm classified as rapid is multiplied by 4, the percent of sperm classified as medium is multiplied by 3, and the percent of sperm classified as slow is multiplied by 2. These values are added together to give the final motility index. (Note that sperm that are classified as static have no value because the index only rates motile sperm.) For example, a semen specimen rated as 42% rapid, 10% medium, 18% slow, and 30% static would have a motility index of 234 ($4 \times 42\% + 3 \times 10\% + 2 \times 18\%$).

Eight hundred and six cycles of IUI from our laboratory (Figure 20.1) demonstrate that couples with a motility index value of 100 or less were less likely to conceive than those whose motility index was above 100.[5] These couples in particular may benefit from media supplementation. This should help explain why the addition of PAF to culture medium may enhance a couple's chance of achieving a pregnancy.[6] Human sperm prepared for IUI using a sperm wash medium supplemented with PAF can result in significantly increased pregnancy rates.[7,8] (Figure 20.2). However, Baka et al.[9] reported that PAF failed to improve IUI pregnancy rates in patients with mild male factor infertility (Figure 20.2), which may be due, in part, to defective PAF receptors.[6] Treatment of sperm in male factor patients with PAF also showed an increase in pregnancy rates.

Additional clinical studies are warranted to further establish the use of PAF therapy for patients undergoing IUI therapy for infertility treatment. In particular, larger numbers of male factor infertility patients will determine the significance of PAF-IUI therapy for these individuals. This may help infertile couples to achieve pregnancy while avoiding more costly and intensive therapies such as *in vitro* fertilization. To summarize, exposure of sperm to PAF during semen washing might significantly increase IUI pregnancy rates (see also Tables 20.1 and 20.2).

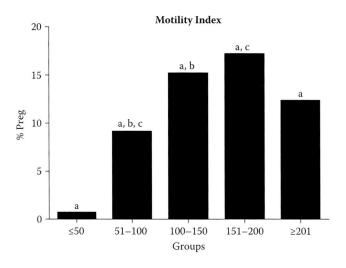

FIGURE 20.1   The likelihood of obtaining a pregnancy through IUI based on motility index. Significantly different: a: $p < 0.01$; b: $p < 0.05$; c: $p < 0.05$.

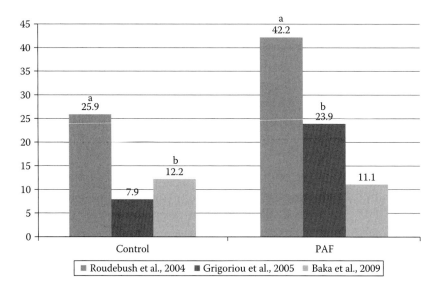

FIGURE 20.2   PAF-IUI pregnancy rates (cumulative). Similar superscripts are significantly different: a: $p < 0.05$; b: $p < 0.05$.

TABLE 20.1

Statements of Chapter 20

Statement	Level of Evidence (LOE)
PAF/IUI improves per cycle and cumulative pregnancy rates in couples with unexplained subfertility	1b

TABLE 20.2

Recommendations of Chapter 20

Recommendation	Grade Strength
PAF might be added to the IUI sperm wash procedure in couples with unexplained subfertility receiving OH/IUI; in couples with male subfertility, more studies are warranted	A

REFERENCES

1. Grassi G., Cappello N., Gheorghe M.F., Salton L., Di Bisceglie C., Manieri C., and Benedetto C. 2010. Exogenous platelet-activating factor improves the motility of human spermatozoa evaluated with C.A.S.A.: Optimal concentration and incubation time. *J Endocrinol Invest* 33(10):684–690.
2. Sengoku K., Tamate K., Takaoka Y., and Ishikawa M. 1993. Effects of platelet-activating factor on human sperm function *in vitro*. *Hum Reprod* 8:1443–1447.
3. Krausz C., Gervasi G., Fori G., and Baldi E. 1994. Effect of platelet activating factor on motility and acrosome reaction of human spermatozoa. *Hum Reprod* 9:471–476.
4. Barratt C.L., Mansell S., Beaton C., Tardif S., and Oxenham S.K. 2011. Diagnostic tools in male infertility—The question of sperm dysfunction. *Asian J Androl* 13:53–58.
5. Lessey, B.A. and Roudebush W.E. 2013. The likelihood of obtaining a pregnancy through intrauterine insemination based on a motility index. Unpublished data.
6. Roudebush W.E. 2007. Seminal platelet-activating factor. *Semin Thromb Hemost* 33(1):69–74.
7. Roudebush W.E., Massey J.B., Toledo A.A., Kort H.I., Mitchell-Leef D., and Elsner C.W. 2004. Platelet-activating factor significantly enhances intrauterine insemination pregnancy rates. *Fertil Steril* 82:52–56.
8. Grigoriou O., Makrakis E., Konidaris S., Hassiakos D., Papadias K., Baka S., and Creatsas G. 2005. Effect of sperm treatment with exogenous platelet-activating factor on the outcome of intrauterine insemination. *Fertil Steril* 83(3):618–621.
9. Baka S., Grigoriou O., Hassiakos D., Konidaris S., Papadias K., and Makrakis E. 2009. Treatment of sperm with platelet-activating factor does not improve intrauterine insemination outcome in unselected cases of mild male factor infertility: A prospective double-blind randomized crossover study. *Urology* 74(5):1025–1028.

21

Oxidative Stress and IUI Outcomes

Alaa Hamada, Ashok Agarwal, and Sergio Oehninger

Introduction

Intra-uterine insemination (IUI) is an assisted reproductive technique (ART) in which washed motile spermatozoa are injected via a catheter into the uterine cavity to fertilize an oocyte. IUI is frequently indicated in several clinical scenarios: cervical hostility, minimal to mild endometriosis, ovarian dysfunction, and infertility (unexplained and male factor). Male factor infertility is the major indication for IUI.

This procedure represents the earliest form of ART and is probably the least effective. However, it is attractive to clinicians because it is relatively simple to perform, inexpensive, and less prone to complications. Many reports recognize that IUI is more effective than timed intercourse (10 to 20% success rate in each cycle). Nevertheless, fertilization failure and unsuccessful pregnancy outcomes are frequently encountered in clinical practice.

A number of factors are responsible for the low pregnancy rates seen with IUI, including oxidative stress. Oxidative stress (OS) occurs when there is excessive generation of reactive oxygen species (ROS) and/or underproduction of protective enzymatic and nonenzymatic antioxidants. ROS, at low levels, are essential for facilitating complex cellular redox interactions and modifying biological molecules, for example, DNA, proteins, and lipids in various cellular organelles. Low levels of ROS can also enhance the ability of human spermatozoa to bind with the zonae pellucida, an effect that is hampered by the addition of the antioxidant vitamin E. Low concentrations of hydrogen peroxide (H_2O_2), when incubated with spermatozoa, can stimulate sperm capacitation and induce spermatozoa to undergo the acrosome reaction. Other types of ROS (e.g., nitric oxide and superoxide anion [O_2]) can also promote sperm capacitation and the acrosome reaction.

Under normal conditions, ROS production is continuously offset by antioxidants that protect biological molecules from being excessively modified, which may lead to their denaturation and aggregation. OS can lead to lipid peroxidation of sperm membrane phospholipids, poor sperm motility due to reduced phosphorylation of axonemal proteins, and defective chromatin packaging and sperm DNA damage. A multitude of OS sources in the IUI setting have been identified (*in vivo* and *in vitro*) from both female and male origins.

There are two types of markers used to evaluate OS in tissues and biological fluids: direct markers such as ROS level, measured by chemiluminescence and total antioxidant capacity, and indirect markers, which are products of oxidation of biological molecules. Malondialdehyde (MDA) results from lipid peroxidation, protein carbonyl results from protein oxidation, and 8-hydroxy-2'-deoxyguanosine, a product of DNA oxidation are examples of indirect markers.

The objective of this chapter is to provide readers with updated information about the role of OS in the IUI setting and whether it has a direct relationship to the IUI outcomes.

Methods

In this chapter we summarize and evaluate the most important and most recent studies examining the role of oxidative stress in IUI and assign level of evidence to these studies (see also Tables 21.1 and 21.2). An extensive literature search was performed using the search engines: PubMed, ScienceDirect, Ovid, and Scopus.

Results

A literature search shows ROS generation in the IUI setting originate from two settings, that is, *in vivo* (from male and female reproductive tracts) and *in vitro* setting (semen processing and use of frozen sperm). Table 21.3 shows the studies that analyzed the IUI outcomes in seminal oxidative stress provoking conditions and or associated conditions. From the male side, leukocytospermia, advanced paternal age, prolonged abstinence time, and high sperm DNA damage are the main conditions which were studied. Antioxidant therapy for male partners shows modest promising effects in improving the IUI cycle outcome.

In the female side, high endometrial content of ROS may explain poor endometrial receptivity and implantation failure observed in women with recurrent IUI cycle failure.

Discussion

Sources of Oxidative Stress in IUI

Male Factors

High Levels of Sperm ROS in In Vivo *Settings*

High levels of seminal ROS are present in 40 to 80% of unselected infertile men.[1] Seminal OS commonly occurs in men with varicocele, leukocytospermia, and/or idiopathic infertility. The main sources of ROS are immature sperm and seminal leukocytes.

High Levels of Sperm ROS in In Vitro *Settings*

A. *Sperm processing methods*—Sperm processing methods are used to obtain highly motile sperm for IUI, and to remove the prostaglandin-rich (induce uterine contraction) and antioxidant-rich seminal plasma. These methods are reported to enhance spermatozoal ROS generation. Dilution and removal of antioxidant-rich seminal plasma and centrifugation employed in double density gradient centrifugation (DDG) result in higher generation of ROS.

B. *Use of frozen sperm*—Cryopreservation can decrease sperm antioxidant activity. Freezing and thawing of equine, human, and bovine sperm has been associated with an increase in ROS generation. Studies using Rhesus Macaque monkeys have shown that frozen-thawed sperm not only experience excessive ROS generation but also contain severe DNA and chromosomal damage. More recently, Gadea et al. reported that total seminal levels of reduced glutathione (GSH) are decreased in human semen that has undergone freezing–thawing cycles.[2]

   A recent study by Kalthur et al. showed that adding antioxidants to cryopreservative medium (e.g., vitamin E) during freezing significantly enhanced post-thaw total motile sperm and the percentage of progressive motility.[3] Such improvements in freezing procedures may ultimately lead to increased conception rates in assisted reproduction. Other authors such as Gadea et al. and Li et al. reported that antioxidants (GSH in the Gadea study and ascorbate and catalase in the Li study) reduce OS markers.[2,4] These findings should encourage companies that produce cryopreservation media to add antioxidants, whether enzymatic or nonenzymatic, to their commercial preparations to enhance post-thaw sperm quality.

TABLE 21.3

Studies Showing IUI Outcomes in Oxidative Stress-Inducing Conditions

Study	Parameters	Patients	Level	Outcomes	Level of Evidence
Milingos, 1996 (Milingos et al., 1996, *Eur J Obstet Gynecol Reprod Biol* 64(1):115–8)	Leukocytospermia	42 couples with repeated IUI failure	Mean 2.9 M/ml	High WBC associated with low PR	2a
Barraud-Lange, 2011 (Barraud-Lange et al., 2011, *Fertil Steril* 96(6):1320–1324)	Leukocytospermia	Artificial insemination of semen in 155 donors and 10,242 infertile men	In donors: 0.8 ± 4.9 M/ml In infertile men: 2.1 ± 16.5 M/ml	High levels of WBC in the semen of donors and infertile men associated with early pregnancy loss and reduced delivery rates	2a
Comhaire, 1995 (Comhaire et al., 1995, *Int J Androl* 18 Suppl 2:76–7)	Leukocytospermia	—	2.3 M/ml	The PR decreased (OR = 0.25, $p<0.05$)	2a
Yang, 2011 (Yang, et al., 2011, *Zhonghua Nan Ke Xue* 17(11):977–83)	Sperm DNA by SCSA	482	DFI >25%	Sperm with DFI >25% had significantly lower PR than those with DFI<OR = 25% (OR: 0.37, 95% CI: 0.14–0.96 and OR: 0.38, 95% CI: 0.16–0.97)	2a
Duran, 2002 (Duran et al., 2002, *Hum Reprod* 17(12):3122–8)	Sperm DNA damage by TUNEL	119 couples undergo 154	Sperm DNA fragmentation >12%	No semen sample with DNA fragmentation >12% resulted in pregnancy	2a
Marshburn, 2010 (Marshburn et al., 2010, *Fertil Steril* (1):286–8)	Abstinence time	866 IUI cycles (372 couples)	<2, <3–5, >5	Higher PR when abstinence ≤2 days	3
Jurema, 2005 (Jurema et al., 2005, *Fertil Steril* 84(3):678–81)	Abstinence time	417 women underwent 929 cycles	≤3, 4 to 10 days	Shorter abstinence time ≤3 days associated with higher PR (14%) vs. 3% in those with >10 days	3
Demir, 2011 (Demir et al., 2011 *J Obstet Gynaecol* 31(5):420–3)	Paternal age	212 infertile couples with 253 cycles	Higher paternal age	Reduced PR	3
Belloc, 2008 (Belloc et al., 2008, *Reprod Biomed Online* 17(3):392–7)	Paternal age	1700 IUI cycles	<30 and >45	Decrease in PR from 12.3% <30 y to 9.3% after 45 y ($p<0.001$) and an increase in miscarriage rate from 13.7% before 30 y to 32.4% after 45 y	3
Mathieu, 1995 (Mathieu et al., 1995, *Hum Reprod* 10(5):1090–7)	Paternal age	901 IUI cycles in 274	Higher paternal age	Decrease in the likelihood of pregnancy ($p = 0.01$)	3

Abbreviations: PR: Pregnancy rate; DFI: DNA fragmentation index.

Seminal OS and IUI Pregnancy Outcomes

Thomson et al. examined levels of 8-hydroxy-2'-deoxyguanosine (8-OHdG)—a biomarker of OS—in the semen of men whose partners were undergoing IUI cycles and reported that levels were significantly lower in those who became pregnant (8.9% versus 20.2% in the non-pregnant women).[5] The authors suggested a threshold value of 11.5% with a sensitivity of 69% and a specificity of 90.9% as a predictor of pregnancy after IUI.[5]

No other study has directly assessed OS markers in relation to IUI outcomes. However, the relationship between seminal OS and IUI pregnancy outcomes can be indirectly inferred from three types of studies:

A. Those that have examined IUI pregnancy outcomes in relation to certain parameters that are linked to OS (see Table 21.3). Certain conditions that are directly linked to OS such as leukocytospermia, sperm DNA fragmentation (usually associated with OS), long abstinence time, and age have been reported to negatively affect IUI pregnancy rates.[6–15]

B. Studies examined the pregnancy outcomes in IUI when male partners were treated with a sort of antioxidant therapy. Treatment of several conditions that are associated with increased seminal OS can improve pregnancy rates in IUI cycles. For example, use of antibiotic and anti-inflammatory therapy (COX-2 inhibitor, rofecoxib) for leukocytospermia, treatment of varicocele, and use of oral antioxidants have been reported to be beneficial in IUI cycles.

Jung et al. reported a successful pregnancy by IUI in a couple after prescribing doxycline and a combination of antioxidants such as vitamin C, E, and zinc for a male partner who had chronic epididymitis and severely impaired spermatogenesis.[16] In a single double blind, randomized trial, Comhaire et al. showed that Astaxanthin 16 mg, a strong antioxidant given to 11 infertile men for 3 months, resulted in a significant reduction in semen ROS and serum Inhibin B levels (LOE 1b).[17] They also reported a significant increase in the sperm linear velocity, in the total, and per cycle pregnancy rates among Astaxanthin group 54.5 and 23.1% versus the placebo cases (10.5 and 3.6%) $P = 0.028$; $P = 0.036$).[17]

Gambera et al. reported a significant improvement in pregnancy rates after IUI (11.3%) and timed intercourse (15.8%) after a 1-month course of rofecoxib (25 mg) for abacterial leukocytospermia (LOE 2b).[18] Furthermore, Daitch et al. reported that when varicocelectomy was performed in 34 men whose female partners underwent IUI cycles afterwards, semen parameters did not significantly improve from preoperative levels.[19] Nevertheless, the pregnancy and live birth rates per cycle were significantly higher in the patients in the varicocelectomy group versus those who did not receive treatment (11.8 versus 6.3% and 11.8 versus 1.6%, respectively) (LOE 2).[19] Although the total motile sperm count was reproducibly reported to affect the IUI outcomes, this clinical scenario suggests that varicocele-induced improvement in sperm function parameters (reduction in the ROS levels and improvement in the sperm DNA integrity), albeit, not specifically measured, may lead to a marked increase in the pregnancy rates with the IUI.

A recent Cochrane meta-analysis on the use of oral antioxidants in male infertility found that these agents significantly improved the assisted (using *in vitro* fertilization and intracytoplasmic sperm injection) and unassisted conception rates and live birth rates and decreased sperm DNA damage (LOE 1a).[20] No clinical trials on IUI were included in this meta-analysis. The improvements in semen parameters were modest, supporting the concept that antioxidants can improve sperm function by improving sperm DNA integrity and fertilizing capabilities.

C. Studies that have examined pregnancy rates in IUI when frozen sperm are used or when semen samples are processed for IUI:

1. *Frozen sperm and IUI outcomes*—Despite the scarcity of well-designed controlled trials on IUI outcomes using frozen sperm, several studies have reported that the fertilizing potential of frozen sperm is lower than that of freshly ejaculated sperm[21] due to cryopreservation-induced sperm dysfunction and OS. Only a single study reported similar pregnancy rates between frozen and freshly ejaculated sperm used in artificial insemination when

there was a sufficient number of progressively motile sperm in the post-thaw specimen and in the absence of severe teratozoospermia and asthenzoospermia.[22]

2. *Sperm processing techniques*—Sperm processing techniques are utilized to prepare a concentrated volume of highly motile sperm. The handling of semen samples during these procedures may result in excessive generation of ROS. There are two commonly used techniques: density-gradient centrifugation (DGC) and swim up. The first technique uses centrifugation to separate fractions of spermatozoa based upon their motility, size, and density. The mature, leukocyte-free spermatozoa are separated from the immature immotile sperm and are then centrifuged. However, the process of centrifugation itself can provoke leukocytes to generate high levels of ROS. Double-density gradient centrifugation is especially associated with high levels of ROS. Reducing the centrifugation time rather than the centrifugation force can minimize the generation of ROS and may assist in retrieval of the highest proportion of mature sperm.

The other technique used to prepare semen for IUI is swim-up technique, in which highly motile sperm are separated based on their natural ability to migrate against gravity. This technique may be inappropriate for semen samples that contain a high concentration of ROS producer cells such as leukocytes, and immature and damaged spermatozoa.

A recent meta-analysis did not find any significant differences in pregnancy rates between these two techniques in the setting of IUI (LOE 1a).[23] However, Ricci et al. showed that the DGC technique resulted in higher recovery rates of total motile, progressive motile, and viable sperm than the swim-up technique.[24] Since the most harmful effects of ROS on sperm are seen in motility and viability, it seems plausible to infer that DGC is associated with the least amount of ROS.[24] Unfortunately, no studies have directly assessed the impact of these techniques on ROS generation and the relationship to IUI outcomes.

Female Factors

Female Reproductive Pathology

Reactive oxygen species are present in the female reproductive tract along with the transcripts of various antioxidant enzymes. Under physiologic conditions, ROS serve as key signal molecules in critical processes such as follicular development, ovarian steroidogenesis, ovulation, corpus luteum formation and luteolysis, decidualization, germ cell function, and early embryo development. On the other hand, OS may affect the efficiency of female reproduction in many ways. In fact, it has been speculated that many reproductive disorders such as endometriosis, embryopathies, preeclampsia, preterm labor, and intra-uterine growth retardation are the result of OS as are prolonged time-to-pregnancy and early pregnancy loss.

IUI has been utilized as adjunct therapy to assist conception in the presence of a variety of female and male pathologies. There are both female and male indications for IUI therapy using the husband's or male partner's sperm (IUIH). These include:

1. Cervical factors (i.e., abnormal mucus production, hostile mucus, presence of anti-sperm antibodies, chronic cervicitis).

2. Coital factors (i.e., reduced frequency, sexual/ejaculatory dysfunctions).

3. Male factors including suboptimal sperm parameters (i.e., male subfertility, such as the presence of mild or moderate oligo-astheno-teratozoospermia or the presence of antisperm antibodies).

4. Unexplained infertility (following a thorough female and male investigation).

5. Relative indications that result in lower pregnancy outcome—this includes endometriosis (minimal or mild, with open tubes) and previously corrected tubal factors (i.e., lysis of mild peri-ovarian and tubal adhesions).[25]

In addition, IUI is the preferred method when artificial insemination using donor sperm (AID) is indicated. In all of these cases, cryopreserved semen/sperm must be used.

Endometrial Receptivity and Oxidative Stress

The germ cells and embryos are vulnerable to the potential harmful effects of ROS, which can arrest embryo development at the two-cell stage. On the other hand, the stromal cells of the endometrium generate ROS as by-products of normal metabolism, and antioxidant enzymes are present in glandular epithelial cells and in stromal cells.

Endometritis, in some animal species, is associated with impaired reproductive performance, possibly due to inflammatory mediators, such as cytokines, eicosanoids, nitric oxide, and OS. An inflammatory milieu in the uterus has been associated with changes in sperm motility and function as well as increased sperm phagocytosis. Furthermore, zygotes resulting from fertilization of oocytes with sperm subjected to OS are less likely to develop into a blastocyst.

Chronic endometritis is a subtle condition that is difficult to diagnose in women. Clinically, the condition is not commonly suspected because chronic endometritis is usually asymptomatic. Also, at hysteroscopy with direct visibility of the endometrial surface, the diagnosis often remains doubtful or unnoticed.

TABLE 21.1

Statements of Chapter 21

Statement	Level of Evidence (LOE)
Lower levels of seminal oxidative stress marker such as 8-hydroxy-2'-deoxyguanosine (8-OHdG) in men whose partners are undergoing IUI cycles is significantly associated with higher pregnancy outcomes	2a
Seminal leukocytospermia is associated with high semen oxidative stress and poor IUI pregnancy outcomes	2a
Factors such as prolonged abstinence time, advanced paternal age which are associated indirectly with high sperm oxidative stress burden are significantly related to poor IUI pregnancy outcomes	3
High sperm DNA damage is associated with low IUI pregnancy rates	2a
Sperm processing methods and use of frozen sperm enhances spermatozoal generation of ROS	2b
The fertilizing potential of frozen sperm is lower than that of freshly ejaculated sperm due to cryopreservation induced sperm dysfunction and OS	1a
Chronic endometritis is associated with impaired female reproductive performance, possibly due to inflammatory mediators, such as cytokines, eicosanoids, nitric oxide, and OS	4

Note: IUI: intrauterine insemination, ROS: reactive oxygen species, and OS: oxidative stress.

TABLE 21.2

Recommendations of Chapter 21

Recommendation	Grade Strength
Oral antioxidants given to infertile men with high semen OS result in significant reduction in semen ROS and serum Inhibin B levels, significant increase in the sperm linear velocity, and in the total, and per cycle IUI pregnancy rates	A
Use of oral antioxidants in male infertility found that these agents significantly improved the assisted (using *in vitro* fertilization and intracytoplasmic sperm injection) and unassisted conception rates and live birth rates and decreased sperm DNA damage	A
Repair of varicocele (condition which produces semen OS) is associated with higher pregnancy and live birth rates per IUI cycle than those who did not receive treatment	C
Use of antibiotic and anti-inflammatory agents for treatment of leukocytospermia is associated with significant improvement in pregnancy rates after IUI	B
Adding antioxidants to cryopreservative medium (e.g., vitamin E) during freezing significantly enhanced post-thaw total motile sperm and the percentage of progressive motility	B
No significant differences in pregnancy rates between the two sperm processing techniques such as density gradient centrifugation (DGC) and swim-up methods in the setting of IUI. DGC technique results in higher recovery rates of total motile, progressive motile, and viable sperm than the swim-up technique	A

A hysteroscopy-guided endometrial biopsy is assumed to be the method of choice when assessing the integrity of the uterine cavity. Although infiltration of the endometrium by lymphocytes and eosinophils is associated with chronic endometritis, the diagnosis is ultimately based on the presence of plasma cells in the endometrial stroma. Even if a histopathological diagnosis is made, the association with OS can be very difficult to establish, and any treatment short of anti-infectious therapy is empirical.

In natural cycles, the luteal phase should be monitored in terms of duration, and occasionally, by measuring mid secretory phase serum progesterone levels. On the other hand, in IUI cycles that are subjected to ovulation induction or augmentation, the luteal phase is typically supplemented with progesterone (usually given by the vaginal route). The role of ovarian hyperstimulation and the resulting hyperestrogenic milieu on gene expression profiles and proteins/molecules key for implantation remains to be clarified.[26]

REFERENCES

1. Lewis S.E., Boyle P.M., McKinney K.A., Young I.S., and Thompson W. 1995. Total antioxidant capacity of seminal plasma is different in fertile and infertile men. *Fertil Steril* October 64(4):868–70.
2. Gadea J., Molla M., Selles E., Marco M.A., Garcia-Vazquez F.A., and Gardon J.C. Reduced glutathione content in human sperm is decreased after cryopreservation: Effect of the addition of reduced glutathione to the freezing and thawing extenders. *Cryobiology* February 62(1):40–6.
3. Kalthur G., Raj S., Thiyagarajan A., Kumar S., Kumar P., and Adiga S.K. 1995. Vitamin E supplementation in semen-freezing medium improves the motility and protects sperm from freeze-thaw-induced DNA damage. *Fertil Steril* March 1;95(3):1149–51.
4. Li Z., Lin Q., Liu R., Xiao W., and Liu W. Protective effects of ascorbate and catalase on human spermatozoa during cryopreservation. *J Androl* September–October 31(5):437–44.
5. Thomson L.K., Zieschang J.A., and Clark A.M. Oxidative deoxyribonucleic acid damage in sperm has a negative impact on clinical pregnancy rate in intrauterine insemination but not intracytoplasmic sperm injection cycles. *Fertil Steril* October 96(4):843–7.
6. Milingos S., Comhaire F.H., Liapi A., and Aravantinos D. 1996. The value of semen characteristics and tests of sperm function in selecting couples for intra-uterine insemination. *Eur J Obstet Gynecol Reprod Biol* January 64(1):115–8.
7. Barraud-Lange V., Pont J.C., Pocate K., Kunstmann J.M., Chalas-Boissonas C., Ducot B. et al. 2011. Seminal leukocytes and clinical outcomes with donor sperm insemination. *Fertil Steril* December 96(6):1320–1324.
8. Comhaire F., Depypere H., and Millingos S. 1995. Statement on intra-uterine insemination. *Int J Androl* December 18 Suppl 2:76–7.
9. Yang X.Y., Zhang Y., Sun X.P., Cui Y.G., Qian X.Q., Mao Y.D. et al. 2011. Sperm chromatin structure assay predicts the outcome of intrauterine insemination. *Zhonghua Nan Ke Xue* November 17(11):977–83.
10. Duran E.H., Morshedi M., Taylor S., and Oehninger S. 2002. Sperm DNA quality predicts intrauterine insemination outcome: A prospective cohort study. *Hum Reprod* December 17(12):3122–8.
11. Marshburn P.B., Alanis M., Matthews M.L., Usadi R., Papadakis M.H., Kullstam S. et al. 2010. A short period of ejaculatory abstinence before intrauterine insemination is associated with higher pregnancy rates. *Fertil Steril* January 93(1):286–8.
12. Jurema M.W., Vieira A.D., Bankowski B., Petrella C., Zhao Y., Wallach E. et al. 2005. Effect of ejaculatory abstinence period on the pregnancy rate after intrauterine insemination. *Fertil Steril* September 84(3):678–81.
13. Belloc S., Cohen-Bacrie P., Benkhalifa M., Cohen-Bacrie M., De Mouzon J., Hazout A. et al. 2008. Effect of maternal and paternal age on pregnancy and miscarriage rates after intrauterine insemination. *Reprod Biomed Online* September 17(3):392–7.
14. Mathieu C., Ecochard R., Bied V., Lornage J., and Czyba J.C. 1995. Cumulative conception rate following intrauterine artificial insemination with husband's spermatozoa: Influence of husband's age. *Hum Reprod* May 10(5):1090–7.
15. Demir B., Dilbaz B., Cinar O., Karadag B., Tasci Y., Kocak M. et al. 2011. Factors affecting pregnancy outcome of intrauterine insemination cycles in couples with favourable female characteristics. *J Obstet Gynaecol* July 31(5):420–3.

16. Jung A., Haidl G., and Schill W.B. 1994. Pregnancy after drug therapy of severe andrological disorder. *Hautarzt* November 45(11):769–71.

17. Comhaire F.H., El Garem Y., Mahmoud A., Eertmans F., and Schoonjans F. 2005. Combined conventional/antioxidant "Astaxanthin" treatment for male infertility: A double blind, randomized trial. *Asian J Androl* September 7(3):257–62.

18. Gambera L., Serafini F., Morgante G., Focarelli R., De Leo V., and Piomboni P. 2007. Sperm quality and pregnancy rate after COX-2 inhibitor therapy of infertile males with abacterial leukocytospermia. *Hum Reprod* April 22(4):1047–51.

19. Daitch J.A., Bedaiwy M.A., Pasqualotto E.B., Hendin B.N., Hallak J., Falcone T. et al. 2001. Varicocelectomy improves intrauterine insemination success rates in men with varicocele. *J Urol* May 165(5):1510–3.

20. Showell M.G., Brown J., Yazdani A., Stankiewicz M.T., and Hart R.J. 2011. Antioxidants for male subfertility. *Cochrane Database Syst Rev* (1):CD007411.

21. Richter M.A., Haning R.V., Jr., and Shapiro S.S. 1984. Artificial donor insemination: Fresh versus frozen semen: The patient as her own control. *Fertil Steril* 1984 February 41(2):277–80.

22. Keel B.A. and Webster B.W. 1989. Semen analysis data from fresh and cryopreserved donor ejaculates: Comparison of cryoprotectants and pregnancy rates. *Fertil Steril* July 52(1):100–5.

23. Boomsma C.M., Heineman M.J., Cohlen B.J., and Farquhar C. 2007. Semen preparation techniques for intrauterine insemination. *Cochrane Database Syst Rev* (4):CD004507.

24. Ricci G., Perticarari S., Boscolo R., Montico M., Guaschino S., and Presani G. 2009. Semen preparation methods and sperm apoptosis: Swim-up versus gradient-density centrifugation technique. *Fertil Steril* February 91(2):632–8.

25. Duran H.E., Morshedi M., Kruger T., and Oehninger S. 2002. Intrauterine insemination: A systematic review on determinants of success. *Hum Reprod Update* July–August 8(4):373–84.

26. Oehninger S. 2008. Revealing the enigmas of implantation: What is the true impact of ovarian hyperstimulation? *Fertil Steril* January 89(1):27–30.

22

Cost-Effectiveness of IUI

Lobke M. Moolenaar, Ben Willem Mol, and Bradley J. Van Voorhis

Introduction

The relative cost-effectiveness of infertility treatments is an important issue. Couples desire infertility treatments that are not only efficacious, allowing for a short time to pregnancy, but also affordable, since infertility care is not a covered benefit in some countries. Although the costs of treatment are often an individual's expense, society, in general, is often burdened by the high costs of caring for premature infants that can result from multiple gestations induced by infertility treatments. Therefore, cost-effectiveness studies are important not only to the individual, but also to the healthcare industry and society. The aim of cost-effectiveness research is to maximize health outcomes with the minimum possible use of resources.

Cost-Effective Infertility Treatments

The most cost-effective approach to an infertile couple will vary depending on the underlying cause of the problem. In some instances, there is little debate about the preferred treatment. For example, in cases of severe tubal disease, the low pregnancy rates after surgery make IVF clearly the treatment of choice from a cost-effectiveness standpoint.[1] Similarly, in a couple presenting with infertility and anovulation, oral ovulation induction medications are effective and inexpensive, making this the logical first line therapy. However, in many other cases, the most cost-effective strategy to infertility care is not as clear. Couples with infertility due to cervical factor, endometriosis, mild to moderate male factor infertility, or unexplained infertility have several options for therapy including intra-uterine insemination (IUI), ovarian hyperstimulation combined with IUI (OH/IUI), or IVF. These treatment options vary considerably in pregnancy rate per cycle and in costs. There are trade-offs to consider with these treatment options as therapies that are more effective generally cost more. Should a couple with unexplained infertility continue trying on their own, attempt conception by IUI, or move directly to IVF? The answer to this question is complex and will depend on the couple's unique circumstances and values. However, costs of treatments and relative effectiveness of the options (the most cost-effective approach) will certainly play an important role in counseling of this couple.

There are several important limitations when evaluating the relative cost-effectiveness of infertility treatments. There have been relatively few large randomized trials of different infertility treatment options, limiting our confidence in comparing effectiveness. On the cost side, many studies have reported infertility treatment charges as a surrogate for the actual cost of providing care. Charges can be artificial and do not necessarily reflect the true costs of providing a service. In addition, the outcome reported by many studies is the cost/delivery of at least one child. This outcome may not include the costs of caring for premature infants—a cost that can be substantial with the high rates of multiple gestations seen with infertility care. On the other hand, from a long-term perspective, twins may "complete" a family for some couples and eliminate the need for future infertility treatments. Finally, cost-effectiveness studies may be based on the outcomes and charges from a few centers limiting the more general applicability of the findings, especially because costs can vary significantly in different countries.

Cost-Effectiveness of Unstimulated IUI and Clomiphene Citrate for Unexplained Infertility

A large, multi-center trial from Scotland compared the outcome of 6 months of unstimulated IUI, clomiphene citrate at a dose of 50 mg for 5 days, and expectant management in couples with 2 years of infertility that was unexplained although women with mild endometriosis and men with sperm motilities as low as 20% were included.[2] Live birth rates were 32/193 (17%) for expectant management, 26/192 (14%) for clomiphene citrate, and 43/191 (23%) for IUI, with none of these being statistically different. Interestingly, couples found active management (IUI or clomiphene citrate) to be more acceptable than expectant management. Not surprisingly, these commonly used empiric treatments were not cost-effective compared to expectant management and raise questions about their use in couples with unexplained infertility.[3] The authors suggested that ovarian stimulation combined with IUI should be the subject of future trials for unexplained infertility as there are differing results in the literature regarding effectiveness.[10,11]

Cost-Effectiveness of IUI, OH/IUI, and IVF

Several retrospective cohort cost-effectiveness studies have compared IUI, OH/IUI, and IVF in couples with a variety of causes of infertility. In light of the prospective randomized study above, these studies are limited in that treatments are not compared to expectant management to know the true incremental benefit of treatment. Moreover, these studies tend to become *dated* as both costs and outcomes change over time. For example, IVF pregnancy rates have increased steadily over time and high-order multiple births have declined as there has been increased emphasis on safety through transfer of fewer embryos. These changes have made IVF a more attractive option since the publication of these studies. Despite these limitations, large cohort studies from individual centers have found IUI alone or IUI with oral ovulation induction to be the most cost-effective first line therapy for couples with infertility due to cervical factor, endometriosis, unexplained infertility, and relatively mild male factor infertility. With more severe abnormalities in semen analysis parameters, IUI is not as effective. Several studies have supported the concept of a threshold value for the total motile sperm count either in the ejaculate (an average of <10 million total motile sperm in at least two samples) or in the postwash inseminate (between 0.8 and 5 million motile sperm) below which IUI becomes significantly less effective. Utilizing these values, there is poor sensitivity for predicting who will conceive with IUI but high specificity for predicting failure to conceive with IUI. For couples with this relatively "severe" male factor infertility, IVF with ICSI appears to be the more cost-effective approach.

Ovarian hyperstimulation can be achieved with oral medications (commonly clomiphene citrate or aromatase inhibitors), gonadotrophin injections, or the combination of both and is frequently combined with IUI for the treatment of infertile couples. A meta-analysis of studies has demonstrated higher pregnancy rates with gonadotrophins as compared to clomiphene citrate, although these medications are more expensive than oral medications.[4] If gonadotrophins are used, the lowest effective doses and careful monitoring of follicular response are required to avoid ovarian hyperstimulation and high-order multiple birth rates due to the use of these medications. The goal of OH should be two mature follicles although despite careful monitoring and dose adjustment, realizing this goal can be difficult. For these reasons, clomiphene citrate is often the first choice for ovarian stimulation before IUI. Some practitioners have chosen to monitor follicular responses by ultrasound with clomiphene citrate to improve timing of the IUI by inducing ovulation with hCG and to monitor for excessive follicular response, although there is no consensus on this practice. The relative cost-effectiveness of OH/IUI and IVF have been the subject of several prospective randomized trials.

Prospective, Randomized Cost-Effectiveness Studies

There have been three prospective randomized trials that have compared IUI (stimulated and unstimulated), OH/IUI, and IVF (Table 22.3). The studies are not directly comparable due to multiple differences

TABLE 22.3

Prospective Randomized Trials Evaluating the Cost-Efffectiveness of IUI

Study	Year	Treatments	N (Couples)	Cost/Cycle	Pregnancy Rate/Cycle	Conclusions
Karande et al.[a]	1999	"Standard care"	50	Not stated		Standard therapy more cost-effective than immediate IVF
		(3 CC-IUI, 3 hMG-IUI, 4 IVF) versus immediate IVF	46		CC-IUI 9.2% hMG-IUI 23.5% IVF 23.9%	
Goverde et al.[b]	2000	IUI alone	86	IUI $298	7.4%	IUI is most cost-effective initial therapy
		hMG-IUI	85	hMG-IUI $446	8.7%	
		IVF	87	IVF $1605	12.2%	
Reindollar et al.[c]	2010	Conventional arm				After initial CC-IUI moving directly to IVF results in lower cost, shorter time to pregnancy
		(CC-IUI X3	247	CC-IUI $500	CC-IUI 7.6%	
		FSH-IUI X3		FSH-IUI $2,500	FSH-IUI 9.8%	
		IVF X6 cycles)		IVF $15,000	IVF 30.7%	
		Accelerated arm	256			
		(CC-IUI X3				
		IVF X6 cycles)				

[a] Karande et al., 1999, *Fertil Steril* 71:468–75.
[b] Goverde et al., 2000, *Lancet* 355:13–18.
[c] Reindollar et al., 2010, *Fertil Steril* 94:888–99

in approach, but they do demonstrate how the cost-effectiveness of various therapies may change as improvements are seen in pregnancy rates with IVF. Karande et al.[9] studied couples with virtually all causes of infertility and compared immediate IVF with a *standard care* algorithm consisting of three cycles of clomiphene citrate-IUI (CC-IUI) followed by three cycles of gonadotrophin injection-IUI (hMG-IUI) followed by up to four cycles of IVF. There were 96 couples randomized to these two treatment arms. There were a number of interesting observations from this study. Thirty two percent of all pregnancies occurred without active treatment in *rest* cycles confirming the observation that couples with infertility can conceive at a reasonably high rate with no therapy at all. Immediate IVF was not a cost-effective approach compared to the *standard* treatment algorithm. Of note, in this relatively small study the pregnancy rate with hMG-IUI was unusually high and was equal to that of IVF. This has not proven to be the case in most other studies as IVF is generally associated with a higher pregnancy rate. The cost analysis in this study was based on full practice charges to the insurance company, which is not necessarily reflective of true costs. In addition, the costs were tracked only until a pregnancy was established but did not include the cost accrued with multiple gestations. Since the multiple gestation rate was quite high in this study, including four sets of triplets, this is an important omission.

Goverde et al.[8] compared three treatment arms of IUI alone, hMG-IUI, and IVF, each performed for up to six cycles in couples with male factor and unexplained infertility. Approximately 85 couples were randomized to each arm of the study. The costs in this study were calculated through 12 weeks after conception and thus did not factor in the high costs associated with multiple gestations. This study found that IUI was as effective as IVF and that OH using injectable gonadotrophins did not yield higher pregnancy rates when combined with IUI. IUI was therefore the most cost-effective first-line therapy for the infertile couple. IUI was also better tolerated by couples as more couples continued with this therapy while IVF was associated with a higher dropout rate. Of note is the extremely low IVF pregnancy rate of 12.2% per cycle, a value which is clearly outdated as compared to modern IVF standards. Nevertheless, the relative cost-effectiveness of IUI was demonstrated with little additional effect seen by adding gonadotrophin stimulation to the treatment prior to IUI. Despite using low doses of FSH (75 IU/ day) and careful monitoring of cycles, the multiple pregnancy rate was 27% in the OH/IUI arm of the study, demonstrating the risky nature of this treatment.

Time to conception is of importance to many couples both to alleviate the suffering and disappointment that comes from being infertile and to avoid the negative effects of aging on their reproductive potential. This factor was recently addressed in a prospective randomized trial termed the Fast Track and Standard Treatment (FASTT) trial.[5] This study enrolled women between the ages of 21 and 39 who had unexplained infertility and a normal ovarian reserve. Male factor infertility was excluded as sperm concentrations of greater than 15 million motile sperm in the ejaculate were required for entry. For this study cost-effectiveness was calculated by summing all insurance charges divided by the number of couples delivering at least one child. Charges were calculated from the time of randomization through hospital discharge of both the mother and baby (-ies) or until one year after the protocol if pregnancy was not achieved. Thus, the cost of multiple gestations and their associated increased hospital perinatal costs were included in this analysis. Out-of-pocket expenses (indirect costs) to the patient were also calculated.

In the study, 243 women were randomized to a *conventional* treatment protocol, which consisted of clomiphene citrate at 100 mg for 5 days plus IUI for three cycles followed by FSH (150 IU/day) stimulated cycles plus IUI for three cycles followed by up to six IVF cycles. Two hundred fifty-six couples were randomized to a *fast track* arm of the study consisting of clomiphene citrate at 100 mg for 5 days plus IUI for three cycles followed immediately by up to six IVF cycles. Fourteen percent of pregnancies were treatment independent occurring in rest cycles. In addition, nearly one fourth of couples were pregnant after the initial three cycles of clomiphene citrate and IUI, demonstrating that this can be a relatively effective therapy in couples with unexplained infertility. If a couple failed to conceive with the initial three cycles of clomiphene citrate-IUI, these authors found that the accelerated arm was (immediate IVF) associated with a shorter time to pregnancy (a median time to pregnancy difference of 3 months) and a lower cost per delivery than patients treated with FSH IUI. The conclusion of this study was that following initial treatment with Clomid and IUI, moving directly to an IVF treatment cycle was the most cost-effective approach for couples with unexplained infertility. Importantly, there were equivalent rates of multiple gestations in the two arms of this study.

Preliminary results of a nationwide cost-effectiveness comparison of OH/IUI using gonadotrophins, natural cycle IVF, and IVF with elective single embryo transfer (INES trial ISRCTN52843371) were recently presented at the ESHRE 2013 meeting. This prospective randomized trial found that OH/IUI was equally effective as these two alternative strategies of IVF had a reasonably low multiple birth rate, and, due to lower per cycle costs, was a more cost-effective strategy for couples with mild male factor or unexplained infertility. In this trial, many treatment-independent pregnancies occurred, raising questions as to when any treatment should be started for these patients with a relatively good prognosis for natural conception.

Conclusions

As we look to the future, it is clear that there may be shifting paradigms as to the most cost-effective treatment strategy for infertile couples. In recent years, there has been a steady increase in pregnancy rates with IVF (see also Tables 22.1 and 22.2). Similar increases have not been achieved with IUI treatments. Indeed, several recent studies modeling outcomes and costs have concluded that moving directly to IVF may be more cost-effective than starting with IUI cycles for unexplained and mild male factor infertility.[6,7] If the singleton delivery rate per cycle can be improved, perhaps with single embryo transfer, IVF may become the favored first-line treatment for most causes of infertility. However, at this time, the balance of prospective randomized trials still favor starting with a more conservative

TABLE 22.1

Statements of Chapter 22

Statement	Level of Evidence (LOE)
Primary treatment with IUI compared to immediate IVF is more cost-effective	1a
In couples with unexplained infertility, treatment-independent pregnancies can occur at a reasonably high rate	1b
IUI with clomiphene citrate followed by IVF improves time to pregnancy compared to IUI with clomiphene citrate followed by IUI r-FSH	1b

TABLE 22.2

Recommendations of Chapter 22

Recommendation	Grade Strength
For couples with unexplained infertility first-line treatment with IUI with clomiphene citrate is cost-effective	A
The use of OH using gonadotrophins and IUI as an intermediate step prior to IVF has to be questioned, although recent data suggests equal efficacy to natural cycle IVF and IVF with elective single embryo transfer	A

treatment regimen of IUI before moving to IVF for the treatment of unexplained infertility. At the same time, the use of OH using gonadotrophin injections and IUI as an intermediate step prior to IVF has to be questioned.

REFERENCES

1. Van Voorhis B.J., Sparks A., Allen B., Stovall D., Syrop C., and Chapler F.K. 1997. Cost–effectiveness of infertility treatment: A cohort study. *Fertil Steril* 67:830–6.
2. Bhattacharya S., Harrild K., Mollison J., Wordsworth S., Tay C., Harrold A., McQueen D., Lyall H., Johnston L., Burrage J., Grossett S., Walton H., Lynch J., Johnstone A., Kini S., Raja A., and Templeton A. 2008. Clomifene citrate or unstimulated intrauterine insemination compared with expectant management for unexplained infertility: Pragmatic randomized controlled trial. *BMJ* 337:a716.
3. Wordsworth S., Buchanan J., Mollison J., Harrild K., Robertson L., Tay C., Harrold A., McQueen D., Lyall H., Johnston L., Burrage J., Grossett S., Walton H., Lynch J., Johnstone A., Kini S., Raja A., Templeton A., and Bhattacharya S. 2011. Clomifene citrate and intrauterine insemination as first-line treatments for unexplained infertility: Are they cost-effective? *Hum Reprod* 26(2):369–75.
4. Cantineau A.E., Cohlen B.J., and Heineman M.J. 2007. Ovarian stimulation protocols (anti-oestrogens, gonadotrophins with and without GnRH agonists/antagonists) for intrauterine insemination (IUI) in women with subfertility. *Cochrane Database Syst Rev* April 18;(2):CD005356.
5. Reindollar R.H., Regan M.M., Neumann P.G., Levine B.S., Thornton K.L., Alper M.M., and Goldman M.B. 2010. A randomized clinical trial to evaluate optimal treatment for unexplained infertility: The fast track and standard treatment (FASTT) trial. *Fertil Steril* 94.888–99.
6. Bhatti T. and Baibergenova A. 2008. A comparison of the cost-effectiveness of *in-vitro* fertilization strategies and stimulated intrauterine insemination in a Canadian health economic model. *J Obstet Gynaecol Can* 30(5):411–20.
7. Pashayan N., Lyratzopoulos G., and Mathur R. 2006. Cost-effectiveness of primary offer of IVF vs. primary offer of IUI followed by IVF (for IUI failures) in couples with unexplained or mild male factor subfertility. *BMC Health Services Research* 6:80.
8. Goverde A.J., McDonnell J., Vermeiden J.P., Schats R., Rutten F.F., and Schoemaker J. 2000. Intrauterine insemination or *in vitro* fertilisation in idiopathic subfertility and male subfertility: A randomised trial and cost-effectiveness analysis. *Lancet* 355:13–18.
9. Karande V.C., Korn A., Morris R., Rao R., Balin M., Rinehart J., Dohn K., Gleicher N. 1999. Prospective randomized trial comparing the outcome and cost of *in vitro* fertilization with that of a traditional treatment algorithm as first-line therapy for couples with infertility. *Fertil Steril* 71:468–75.

10. Guzick. D.S., Carson, S.A., Coutifaris, C., Overstreet, J.W., Facfor-Litrak, P., and Steinkompf, M.P. 1999. Efficacy of superovulation and intrauterine insemination in the treatment of infertility. National Cooperative Reproductive Medicine Network. *N Engl J Med* 340:177–83.

11. Steures. P., van der Steeg, J., Hompes, P., Habbema, J., Eijkemans, M., Broekmans, F., Verhoeve, H., Bossuyt, P., van der Veen, F., and Mol, B. 2006. Intrauterine insemination with controlled ovarian hyperstimulation versus expectant management for couples with unexplained subfertility and an intermediate prognosis: A randomized clinical trial. *Lancet* 368:216–21.

23

Minimal Standards and Organization for Donor Sperm Banking

Nicolás Garrido and Antonio Pellicer

Objectives Pursued by the Donation

With sperm donation, couples and practitioners are pursuing the achievement of a healthy newborn with the maximum likelihood to succeed while also minimizing risk of transmission of infectious and genetic diseases or other undesired medical conditions (GS: Grade Strength of each Recommendation, see Table 23.2) (GS-D). In developing countries, this should be complemented with a cautious cost/benefit evaluation, mainly based on existing evidence and accurate risk estimation.

Even though this should be the goal of each assisted reproduction provider and also the desire of every single woman or couple, under a global perspective there are wide regional differences due to the different legal, social, and demographic conditions on the application of such donation programs (GS-D).

The aim of our work is to define the minimum requirements to implement a sperm donation program, focusing on developing countries having limited resources, stressing the justified investments while alleviating all the unnecessary assets, based on a literature review of the existing evidence.

Minimal Requirements to Constitute a Sperm Bank

Technical and Lab Resources

The minimal technical requirements and devices needed to run a donor sperm bank from scratch, apart from the proper building where a laboratory is going to be placed, with all the architectural requirements depending on local regulations, will include all the resources to enable the selection of donors, including the place to conduct personal interviews, filing, semen analyses, and also the capacity to store and maintain frozen sperm samples, meaning that the proper containers and a continuous supply of refrigeration must be guaranteed.

Also, there is the need for the equipment required to perform blood, urine, and semen tests to confirm the absence of infectious and genetic conditions, although all these may be replaced by an adequate referral to external laboratories (GS-D).

In this sense, the minimal shopping list should include:

1. Laminar flow hoods and incubators, with CO_2 supply in order to receive, let liquefaction run properly, maintain and handle sperm samples mimicking also the natural situation, under the most sterile conditions available.
2. Bright-field microscopes in order to analyze the samples, as well as centrifuges to concentrate sperm cells from a raw ejaculate, that will be needed in some cases.
3. Nitrogen tanks where the samples will be kept frozen until future use, with periodical supply, ensuring that the freezing chain is not broken.

4. Ideally, an electronic filing system, or at least a paper-based filing system, to keep all donor records available.

5. There is also a need to have reference laboratories, in order to perform the screening tests for both infectious and genetic disorders, if these are not going to be run at the sperm bank facility.

6. Additionally, there is an obligation to generate and maintain standard operational procedures for each procedure, as well as records about regular maintenance and repair of all the equipment.

Moreover, the qualified and trained personnel in an assisted reproduction laboratory, including cryobiology, quality assessment, serological, and genetic tests are required as lab directors and technical personnel.

Safety

Sperm Donor Selection

The most relevant issue to constitute a donor sperm bank relies on the process to select sperm donors. The main qualities to seek when evaluating potential donors are: first, an assurance of good psychophysical health status with confirmed absence of transmissible infectious and genetic conditions, and second, having an optimal sperm quality (GS-D).

In fact, given the likelihood of rejecting potential donors and the costs, it should be performed exactly in the opposite way: first, confirming sperm quality above the established thresholds (where there is a rejection rate of approximately 70–80% of the candidates), and then, the clinical history, exams, and tests.

These goals may be attained by means of a careful anamnesis together with a battery of tests, and adequate risk management and information to the patients. There is no "right formula" to select donors, given that several genetic diseases may not be evident (or even known by the donor, for instance, carrying recessive conditions), and unexpected transmission of these is a real possibility (LOE: Level of Evidence of each Statement, see Table 23.1 LOE 4).

Donor Anamnesis: Medical History and Physical Examination

Regarding the medical and surgical history, donors should declare that they are healthy and give no history suggesting potentially transmissible diseases.[1-4]

A complete genetic history from him and his family is mandatory, and the donor should not declare that he has any major inheritable condition, such as familial diseases with a main genetic component, such as cleft lip or palate, congenital hip dislocation, clubfoot, hypospadias nor any significant Mendelian disorder (albinism, hemophilia, hemoglobin disorders, neurofibromatosis), or with known or related genetic component: for example, debilitating asthma, juvenile diabetes mellitus, epileptic disorder, and so forth (GS-D).

Usually, depending on the ethnical background, some genetic diseases are recommended to be investigated in the donors, such as being heterozygous for an autosomal recessive gene, for example, cystic fibrosis, glucose-6-phosphate dehydrogenase deficiency or ß-thalassemia, sickle cell, Tay–Sachs disease. Then, the list of genetic tests should be objectively customized depending on the prevalence of the different diseases among the donor's origin and the cost/benefit evaluation (GS-D).

Only in exceptional circumstances (known donation, where allowed) these may not necessarily be avoided, provided that all parties are fully informed and supervised by qualified clinical geneticists. Although not permitted in some countries, other accepts having donors with a known recessive condition if patients accept and the female has been found to be negative for the same.[3]

This obviously leads to rejection of candidates who declare that they have been adopted or have unknown familiar origin, since their unknown genetic history impedes this investigation (GS-D).

On the other hand, a complete personal and sexual history should be obtained to identify individuals who might be at high risk for infections potentially transmissible via gamete donation, with high risk behaviors, and also lifestyle issues that may be affecting sperm quality, or inducing a risk to the recipients or offspring.[3,4] For these, rejection as donors or increased testing frequency should be considered (GS-D).

For instance, having a history of previous STIs (e.g., genital warts or have been treated for syphilis, gonorrhea, or chlamydia within the preceding year), unprotected intercourse and multiple partners may help to identify *high-risk candidates* (LOE 4).

Following some international recommendations, based on the correlation between some behaviors and higher incidence of such diseases, those men who had sex with another man in the recent past, had injected drugs for nonmedical reasons, have received human-derived clotting factor concentrates, who have had sex in exchange for money or other compensations, or having sex in the preceding year with any person meeting any of the criteria described before, and even those incarcerated should be included within this group (GS-D).[3]

Also, those having been in contact with an open wound, nonintact skin, or mucous membrane to blood that is known or suspected to be infected with HIV, hepatitis B, and/or hepatitis C virus, and even close contact with these persons one year preceding the donation are included. Receiving a blood transfusion or any medical treatment that involved blood transfusion, xenotransplants, received human organs, or human extracts should be also carefully and regularly screened. Transmissions of Creutzfeldt–Jakob disease, West Nile virus, and a quarantine period after smallpox vaccination have been considered by American regulations, although there are no evidences of their effects as STDs (GS-D).[3]

Regarding the age limit, the evidence of its effect on the offspring are highly controversial (LOE 2a), and have been related with increased risk of very infrequent conditions, such as new mutations of the paternal genome involving achondroplasia, autism, dyskinetic cerebral palsy, multiple sclerosis, oral clefts, retinoblastoma, schizophrenia, increased aneuploidy in the fetus, and also increased risk of miscarriage.

The donor should be of legal age and, ideally, less than 40 years of age, because increased male age is associated with a progressive increase in the prevalence of aneuploid sperm (LOE 2a), although for known donation a higher limit is acceptable if the recipients agree to the increased genetic risk. In these cases, the recipients should be offered the possibility of prenatal diagnosis if a pregnancy occurs (GS-D).[3,4]

Selection of donors with established fertility is desirable but not required. In our experience, all donors with sufficient sperm samples have been able to obtain newborns with the use of assisted reproduction technologies.

Physical examination is also convenient, and every 6 months while remaining an active donor, carried out by an appropriately trained clinician to assist in the detection of inherent congenital abnormalities (e.g., hypospadias), seeking for physical evidence of risk of sexually transmitted disease such as genital ulcerative lesions, herpes simplex, chancroid, or urethral discharge, syphilis, evidence of anal intercourse including perianal condylomata, urethral discharge or genital warts indicating a possible infection of papilloma virus or herpes simplex virus, and also evidence of high-risk behavior such as nonmedical percutaneous drug use (needle tracks, tattoos, piercings, etc.), as well as disseminated lymphadenopathy, unexplained oral thrush and spots consistent with Kaposi sarcoma, unexplained jaundice, hepatomegaly, or icterus, as well as eczema vaccinatum, generalized vesicular, rash, and severely necrotic lesion (GS-D).

Sexually Transmitted Diseases Testing

Taking as reference the standards established by the European Union Tissues Directive, each country may include strict requirements regarding the infectious diseases to be screened in potential donors, as the U.S. Food and Drug Administration also states (GS-D).[1–4] These requirements may be less rigorous than those in the state in which an individual practice is located, or than those recommended by the American Society for Reproductive Medicine (ASRM) and the Society for Assisted Reproductive Technology (SART).

The screening of donors before acceptance should include, but not be limited to tests enabling the ruling out of the presence of:

HIV-1 and -2

Hepatitis C

Hepatitis B (both surface antigen and core antibody)

Serologic test for syphilis

HTLV-1 and HTLV-2 (depending on the donor's origin)

CMV (IgG and IgM). In locations where the prevalence of CMV-seropositive men without active infection is high (leading to discarding many potential donors), their acceptance and use in also CMV seropositive female partner is permissible, although the practice is not entirely without risk, because there are many strains of CMV and superinfection is possible.

Semen, urine, or a urethral swab should be obtained to test for *Neisseria gonorrhoeae* and *Chlamydia trachomatis* (GS-D).

Additional testing not required by the FDA but recommended by the ASRM may include blood type and Rh to adequately match the donor with the recipients' group, avoiding the resulting newborn with a blood type not possible from the parents' combination, and also Rh incompatibility with the mother, where couples should be informed about obstetric significance of this condition (GS-D).

Before sperm samples can be used, the need to repeat these tests every 6 months arises, in order to keep quarantine and surpassing silent window periods, mainly for HIV infections. Expensive techniques based on nucleic acids could diminish this time range (GS-D).

The frequency at which tests need to be repeated will depend on the frequency of the samples released by the donor, and the number of samples that will be released with the tests' results, combined with the stock of samples available, and the risk of the donor to seroconvert.

For instance, repeated serologies may be requested in high-risk donors, or those whose samples are immediately needed for use, while longer periods may be established in donors when their samples are not frequently employed, or providing few samples per month (thus releasing a low number of samples per month and per test) (GS-D).

What to Do with the Screening Results Available

If testing is negative at the time of donor selection, semen samples may be collected and prepared for cryopreservation.

A positive test should be verified before notifying the potential donor. If a test is confirmed positive, the individual should be referred for appropriate counseling and management (GS-D).

Individuals who initially test positive for syphilis, *Neisseria gonorrhoeae*, or *Chlamydia trachomatis* should be treated, retested, and deferred from donation for 12 months after documentation that treatment was successful before being reconsidered. If evidence is presented that treatment occurred more than 12 months ago and was successful, no further deferral is needed as long as current testing does not indicate an active infection.

Other positive results make donors not eligible for anonymous donation.[1-4]

After donation, anonymous donor specimens must be quarantined for a minimum of 180 days. The donor must be retested after the required quarantine interval, and specimens may be released only if the results of repeat testing are negative (GS-D).

Genetic Testing (General and Ethnically Oriented)

Genetic screening for heritable diseases should be performed in potential sperm donors. It is interesting to remark that there is no sperm without a risk, and it is estimated that all people will carry a mean of 5–10 recessive mutations (LOE 3), this being only a problem if that person's partner (or the receiver of donated sperm) carries a mutation in the same gene.

Then, there is no correct decision about the list of genetic conditions to be tested, it being the international recommendation to determine the most prevalent among the donor's and patient's origin, and discuss with the patients about the need to test (GS-D).

In this sense, potential donors should ordinarily screen negative for the following conditions according to their ethnic background and prevalence:

Cystic fibrosis (e.g., Caucasian)

Beta-thalassemia (e.g., Mediterranean, Middle East, Indian subcontinent)

Sickle cell disease (e.g., African and Afro-Caribbean)

Tay–Sachs disease (e.g., Jews of Eastern European descent)

In exceptional circumstances (known donation, depending on local regulations), donors who screen positive may be accepted after consultation with an appropriately qualified clinical geneticist or consultant hematologist (as appropriate) (GS-D).

The list of genetic tests can be increased, depending on the donor's origin, and also (most frequently) in the cases of patients where a female recessive condition has been determined. Then, the donor can be tested specifically for this condition, in order to avoid the transmission of this particular genetic disease.

Karyotyping

All donors should be screened, since the frequency of balanced translocations is around 2 per 1,000 tested individuals (LOE 2a), and some cytogenetic abnormalities have been detected during screening of sperm donors, while the actual costs of a karyotype can be affordable.

A donor found to have a significant chromosomal abnormality should be rejected (GS-D).

Psychological Testing

Implication counseling by a qualified mental health professional is recommended strongly for all sperm donors at the time of recruitment before screening in order to protect the recipient and the future child (GS-D).

Regarding the recipient, the potential impact of the relationship between the donor and recipient should be analyzed as well as the potential psychological risks and information about the extent of information about him to be disclosed now or later.

Regarding the newborn, psychological evaluation of the general abilities and intellectual capacity of the donor candidates is necessary to permit detection of potentially inheritable mental disorders or at least those with a relevant genetic component (GS-D).

Issues Related to Sperm Freezing and Banking

For several decades sperm cells have been successfully frozen to be employed afterwards. This allowed a wide and worldwide experience regarding the main concerns when establishing a tissue bank to be addressed by evaluating the experience retrospectively (GS-D).

We can divide the safety items linked to the establishment of a sperm bank into those involving the operators, the sperm samples, and also the patients being treated with previously cryopreserved samples.

All the operators from a sperm bank should be aware and take the appropriate measures to mitigate the risks, mainly those concerning N_2 handling that may result in skin burn and eye harm due to spill and contact, and also the possibility of inhalation of N_2 vapors that may inadvertently cause a decrease in O_2 concentration, leading to loss of consciousness, cerebral harm, and even death (LOE 2a). Then, control of oxygen levels, and the use of adequate self-protection materials such as glasses and gloves is required (GS-D).

More infrequently, reports of cryovials and even tank explosions have been reported; the latter can be avoided by a frequent revision of the tank valves.

Regarding the risks involving the adequate maintenance of sperm samples, they mainly concern the loss/damage of material, and also involve misidentification. To this end, the proper methods to confirm all the information related to the samples and their storage should be implemented, together with the systems avoiding the material losses, including the fall to the bottom of the tank, or even a tank breakage, involving the loss of all samples.

Then, routine supervision is obligatory, and the implementation of surveillance systems and emergency plans are advised.

About the patients' risks, we can divide them into those involving the transmission of undesired consequences to the offspring or receivers: first are the risks linked to the freezing/procedure itself, and second are the risks associated with the storage system. The first is in regard to the wide experience and lack of a described relationship between the use of frozen sperm samples using classic freezing with any alteration on embryo quality and even the offspring conceived (LOE 3). Regarding the second, there has never been described a single case of cross-contamination of reproductive tissues stored within the same tanks, even after uncountable spermatozoa have been stored for many years throughout the entire world (LOE 3).

Nevertheless, the European Parliament and Council has published its Directive 2004/23/EC on setting the standards of quality and safety for the donation, procurement, testing processing, preservation, storage, and distribution of human tissues and cells.

The aim of this regulation involving reproductive cells is to safeguard public health and prevent the transmission of infectious diseases, from their donation, up to their use, also aiming to unify the European standards. Nevertheless, it also recognizes the possibility of causing unwanted effects and diseases, even after being evaluated.

Efficacy

Fertility Tests in the Sperm Donors

Semen analysis, as stated by the World Health Organization, is up to now the only worldwide accepted tool to diagnose male fertility; however, its predictive value to assess male capacity to initiate a pregnancy is relatively low (LOE 2a).

With the introduction of *in vitro* fertilization and especially intracytoplasmatic sperm injection, the fertility problems caused by a diminished sperm production were frequently solved, but the secrets of sperm physiology still remained undiscovered.

Moreover, a high percentage of males with apparently normal semen are not able to impregnate a normal healthy woman during her reproductive life (LOE 2a), so improvements in the diagnostic tools to accurately assess male fertility potential are necessary. Then, the only tool to assess male fertility will be the measurement of the total number of motile spermatozoa within a single ejaculate (GS-D), but there are no uniformly accepted standards, but, in general, the minimum criteria for normal semen quality can be applied.[5]

Our recommendation in this sense is to select donors to consider that the need to freeze, maintain quarantined, and thaw sperm samples will take approximately 60% of all motile sperm in the raw ejaculate, and the number of motile sperm to maximize (IUI) likelihood to succeed is 2 million. To reach these levels, the number of motile sperm after thawing needs to reach 15 million.

This clearly points to the fact that ejaculates below 40 million of total motile sperm are unlikely to achieve these thresholds, thus not being able to prepare intra-uterine insemination (IUI). Every number above 40 million will increase each ejaculate's profitability, combined with the adequate freezing protocols enabling partial thawing of the samples, depending on the needs (IUI or IVF) and the post-thawing test results. For semen quality testing, it is suggested that 2 to 3 samples be examined (each after a 2- to 5-day abstinence interval) before proceeding with a more extensive evaluation.

Results to Be Expected/Obtained with Donor Sperm IUI

From our experience in more than 3,000 donor IUI and IVF (57 and 42.8%, respectively), from several centers among our group, the results to be expected are around 23% pregnancy rates in IUI using mild ovarian hyperstimulation, since in nonobstructive azoospermia patients presented the highest (29.1%) compared with cases of ICSI failure and single women (27.6 and 22.6%, respectively). Pregnancy rates in IVF using donor sperm are around 45%, where couples with previous ICSI failures exhibited the highest pregnancy rates in IVF cycles (48.7%) compared with azoospermia and single women groups (42.0 and 38.2%, respectively) (LOE 3).

Conditions of Use: Anonymity and Compensation

Some general remarks on the use of donor sperm should also be introduced, aiming to avoid future inconveniences, even thinking that these issues can fall beyond regulations.

First, the number of newborns obtained from each donor should be carefully considered, and an exact number is extremely difficult to justify. In this sense, too many increase the likelihood of unaverted consanguinity in the future, although several epidemiological studies demonstrate that this is less probable than averted consanguinity (LOE 3). Moreover, nondonor parenthood is not controlled in this way.

In contrast, having an extremely low number of children per donor will substantially decrease the cost/benefit ratio of the assets invested, thus there is the risk of an increased cost per donor, making difficult the implementation of these programs.

No owner, operator, laboratory director, or employee may serve as a donor in that practice, neither the patient's physician nor the individual performing the actual insemination can be the sperm donor (GS-D).

TABLE 23.1

Statements of Chapter 23

Statement	Level of Evidence (LOE)
The donor should be of legal age and, ideally, less than 40 years of age, because increased male age is associated with a progressive increase in the prevalence of aneuploid sperm	2a
The results to be expected are around 23% pregnancy rates in IUI using mild ovarian hyperstimulation; pregnancy rates in IVF using donor sperm are around 45%	3
Unexpected transmission of genetic diseases using donor sperm is a real possibility	4
All donors should be screened for karyotype, since the frequency of balanced translocations is around 2 per 1,000 tested individuals	2a
Inhalation of N_2 vapors may inadvertently cause a decrease in O_2 concentration, leading to loss of consciousness, cerebral harm, and even death	2a

TABLE 23.2

Recommendations of Chapter 23

Recommendation	Grade Strength
With sperm donation, couples and practitioners are pursuing the achievement of a healthy newborn with the maximum likelihood to succeed while also minimizing risk of transmission of infectious and genetic diseases or other undesired medical conditions	D
The main qualities to seek when evaluating potential donors are: first an assurance of good psycho-physical health status with confirmed absence of transmissible infectious and genetic conditions, and second, having an optimal sperm quality	D
Taking as reference the standards established by the European Union Tissues Directive, each country may include strict requirements regarding the infectious diseases to be screened in potential donors, as the U.S. Food and Drug Administration also states	D
A complete genetic history from the donor and his family is mandatory, and the donor should not declare that he does not have any major inheritable condition	D

REFERENCES

1. E.U. Directive 2004/23/EC. 2004. Directive of the European Parliament and of the Council of 31 March 2004 on setting standards of quality and safety for the donation, procurement, testing, processing, preservation, storage and distribution of human tissues and cells. *J Eur Union* 102:48–58.
2. E.U. Directive 2006/17/EC. 2006. Implementing Directive 2004/23/EC of the European Parliament and of the Council as regards certain technical requirements for the donation, procurement and testing of human tissues and cells. *J Eur Union* 38:40–52.
3. Practice Committee of American Society for Reproductive Medicine; Practice Committee of Society for Assisted Reproductive Technology. 2008. Guidelines for gamete and embryo donation: A Practice Committee report. *Fertil Steril* November 90(5 Suppl):S30–44.
4. ESHRE Task Force on Ethics and Law. 2002. Gamete and embryo donation. *Hum Reprod* May 17(5):1407–8.
5. World Health Organization. 2010. *Laboratory Manual for the Examination of Human Semen*, 5th ed. Geneva, Switzerland: World Health Organization.

24

Indications for Donor Sperm Including Lesbian Couples and Single Women

Anne Brewaeys

Introduction

Although there is an increase in lesbian and single mothers applying at fertility clinics, the acceptance of these requests remains controversial in some fertility centers. This article reviews the current empirical knowledge about mother–child relationships and child development in lesbian and single mother families.

Single and lesbian mothers feature a number of similarities and differences that might influence family development. The most controversial characteristic of both family types is *the absence of a father*. In most societies the fundamental conviction prevails that a father is essential for healthy psychological development. Children growing up without a male parental figure would be at risk for identity confusion. Furthermore, in both family types the absent father is replaced by a *sperm donor*. Thus, all children will be unknown with half of their genetic makeup. In contrast with heterosexual donor insemination (DI) families where the donor origin is often kept a secret, children of lesbian and single mothers are aware of their donor conception in an early developmental stage.

Although they have the absence of a father (figure) in common, two essential differences remain between lesbian and single mothers. Lesbian women applying for DI intend to raise their child together with their female partner. In contrast with single mothers, their child will grow up with two parents instead of one. Sharing educational tasks with a partner is different from doing it alone. Being a single parent might induce extra stress for mother and child. On the other hand, single mothers appear to be mainly heterosexual, thus their children will not have to deal with their mothers' homosexuality and with potential homophobic reactions.

Empirical Follow-Up Studies

Single Mother Families

Since the number of single mother families has dramatically increased in western society, data of several population studies have become available. Results are unanimous. Mothers perceive more parental stress; have more psychological and physical health problems. When the children are compared with children raised in two parent families they appear to have more problems on all variables involved: psychopathology, cognitive development, socio-emotional development, and the ability to engage in intimate relationships. However, a number of crucial differences between the families mentioned above and mothers who have planned to become a single parent by means of DI make the results inappropriate for the latter group. The majority of children in previous studies experienced parental separation and the single parent never intended to raise a child on her own. As it is well known that parental conflict and divorce have a negative impact on children, these data tell us little about DI children and mothers who were single by choice.

Single Mothers by Choice

Who are those single women who want a child by means of a sperm donor and what do we know about their children? Studies remain sparse, samples are small and not always representative. Most children studied were younger than 5 years and belonged to white, socially privileged families. Consequently, crucial questions about the quality of life of adolescents and adults raised in a diversity of social contexts have not yet been addressed.

Motives and Demographic Features

All interviewed women were aware of their biological clock, which did not allow any further delay of their child project. Their mean age when applying at the fertility clinic appeared to be higher than 35 years. The majority of women were highly educated. Most of these women went through a period of grief for not having found the appropriate partner at the appropriate moment. So, becoming a single DI mother was not their first choice.[1,2]

Psychological, Relational, and Social Characteristics

Mothers were psychologically healthy and could rely on a supportive social and family network, all had had meaningful partner relationships in the past.[1,2] What these findings do not tell us is why they failed to build a family with their previous partners. Did some of these women lack the abilities to develop long lasting intimate relationships or is it the changing social context that makes it hard for some well-educated women to find the right man?

Family Relationships and the Psychological Development of Children

When compared with two-headed heterosexual families, no major differences were found in the *quality of mother–child relationships*. However, single mothers appeared to be more emotionally involved with their child and felt more satisfied with being a mother. Child development was similar in both family types. The social, cognitive, emotional, and behavioral development of the children did not differ.[2,3] One must keep in mind that children were still young. One recent study of adults raised in single mother families revealed the following findings: overall, quality of parenting and psychological adjustment was similar compared with two-headed heterosexual families. Where differences were identified between family types, these pointed toward more positive family relationships and greater well-being in the single mother families.[4]

Lesbian Mother Families

There is these days a considerable body of knowledge on lesbian mothers and their children (for review see Bos et al.[5] and Tasker[6]). The design and research questions changed over the years and a brief overview will be presented. The first studies were carried out among children of postdivorced lesbian mothers who came out as homosexuals after the birth of their child.[7] More than 10 years later, when the first lesbian couples started to apply at fertility clinics, new studies emerged.[8] In previous lesbian families, all children had a known father, thus now researchers investigated what it meant for children to be fatherless right from birth. When it appeared from studies carried out so far that the still very young children were doing fine, there was a growing need for knowledge about adolescents and adults of lesbian mothers. Indeed, young children do not have the cognitive and emotional abilities to fully understand the special features of their family. And it is only during adolescence that they fly out in the often homophobic world. Only a few longitudinal studies were carried out in which grown-up children themselves were questioned about having a lesbian mother.[4,9,10,11]

Despite the differences in research designs, number of participants, and used instruments, findings were strikingly unanimous. With regard to the *development of family relationships* during childhood and adolescence, lesbian mothers did not differ in the quality of the parent–child relationships compared with heterosexual DI and naturally conceived families. They were equally emotionally involved and equally disciplined the child. Grandparents did accept these children as their offspring.

However, a number of interesting differences with the heterosexual family did appear. The comother, the biological mother's lesbian partner, was more involved in all aspects of child rearing than the heterosexual father and educational tasks were more equally divided between lesbian mothers than between mothers and fathers in the heterosexual families. The *psychological development* of children raised by lesbian mothers was similar in all studies. Children were well adjusted and showed normal emotional, behavioral, and social development. Only a few studies investigated the gender role development of lesbian mother's offspring, and they failed to find any difference compared with children of heterosexual families. However, children were often too young to fully investigate their sexual orientation. All these findings are pretty reassuring and one wonders whether children experience any homophobic reaction in their social surroundings. Two studies investigated this issue in detail. Children became more secretive about their nontraditional family when growing older and they appeared to be more selective to whom they disclosed their two-mother family unit.[10] In the U.S. study by Gartrell and colleagues, nearly half had experienced some form of homophobia and those who did reported more psychological distress.[11]

Children's Donor Concept

Children of lesbian and single mothers are informed about the use of a donor in an early developmental stage and this is in sharp contrast with the majority of heterosexual parents. Once these youngsters reached adolescence, the majority were curious about certain donor characteristics such as physical and personality traits. At least half of them wanted to meet the donor. Whether or not children were conceived by an anonymous or identity registered donor seemed to make only a small difference in their curiosity.[9,11,12]

Discussion

A brief overview was presented of the most relevant empirical findings with regard to family relationships and child development in single and lesbian mother families. The sparse studies investigating single women applying in fertility clinics outlined a picture of last chance mothers not wanting to wait any longer for an appropriate partner. Overall, these women were highly educated and had a supportive social network. Although minor differences had been identified between single mother and two parent families, no major negative effect was found on family relationships and child development (see Tables 24.1 and 24.2). Findings remain preliminary and the majority of children involved were of preschool age. Questions about emotional, social, and identity development during adolescence and adulthood remain. Large-scale longitudinal studies are still needed.

In contrast with the former group, there is a larger body of evidence about lesbian mother families and no adverse effect of lesbian motherhood could be identified. Family relationships were stable and children were doing well. The majority of adolescents were curious about certain donor characteristics and a respectable number wanted to meet him. What we do not know is if the absence of a father figure influenced their curiosity. Studies of adults raised in a lesbian family remain sparse. Therefore, findings about the sexual orientation of lesbian mother's offspring remain inconclusive. Another issue also needing more attention is the effect of social stigmatization. One should realize that the families studied were privileged: mothers were white, well educated, and living in a tolerant social environment. Replication studies in a diversity of social contexts are needed.

Based on the empirical findings so far, these women should not be excluded from DI programs. Just like heterosexual DI applicants they fare well with appropriate counseling that addresses their specific characteristics and needs. Taking into account that the majority of their children wishes (identifying) donor information, the use of identity registered donors is strongly advised. However, the reader must keep in mind that the impact of empirical research findings remains relative compared with the role of cultural, religious, and moral values. Consequently, the well-being of these families is colored by the degree of tolerance in their specific social context.

TABLE 24.1

Statements of Chapter 24

Statement	Level of Evidence (LOE)
Family relationships and psychological development of children are normal	3
Social stigmatizations influence well-being of family members negatively	3
Most children want (identifying) donor information	3

TABLE 24.2

Recommendations of Chapter 24

Recommendation	Grade Strength
Single and lesbian women should be accepted in DI programs when professional counseling is available	D
The use of identity registered donors is strongly advised	D

REFERENCES

1. Leiblum S., Palmer M., and Spector I. 1995. Nontraditional mothers: Single heterosexual and lesbian couples electing motherhood via donor insemination. *J Psychosom Obstet Gynecol* 15:11–20.
2. Murray C. and Golombok S. 2005. Going it alone: Solo mothers and their infants conceived by donor insemination. *American Journal of Orthopsychiatry* 75:242–253.
3. MacCallum F. and Golombok S. 2004. Children raised in fatherless families from infancy. *J Child Psychology and Psychiatry* 45:1407–1419.
4. Golombok S. and Badger S. 2010. Children raised in mother-headed families from infancy: A follow up of lesbian and single heterosexual mothers, at early adulthood. *Human Reprod* 25:150–157.
5. Bos H.M., van Balen F., and van den Boom D.C. 2005. Lesbian families and family functioning: An overview. *Patient Educ Couns* 59:263–275.
6. Tasker F. 2010. Same sex parenting and child development: Reviewing the contribution of parental gender. *J of Marriage and Family* 72.35–40.
7. Golombok S. 1983. Children in lesbian and single parents households. *J Child Psychol Psychiatr* 38:783–791.
8. Brewaeys A., Ponjaert I., Van Hall E., and Golombok S. 1997. Donor Insemination: Child and family development in lesbian-mother families with children of 4-to 8 years old. *Human Reprod* 12:1349–1359.
9. Vanfraussen K., Ponjaert I., and Brewaeys A. 2001. An attempt to reconstruct children's donor concept: A comparison between children's and lesbian parents' attitudes towards donor anonymity. *Human Reprod* 16:2019–2025.
10. Vanfraussen K., Ponjaert-Kristoffersen I., and Brewaeys A. 2002. What does it mean for youngsters to grow up in a lesbian family created by means of donor insemination? *J Reproductive and Infant Psychology* 20, 4:237–254.
11. Gartrell N., Deck A., Rodas C., Peyser H., and Banks A. 2005. The national lesbian family study 4. Interviews with the 10 year old children. *Am J Orthopsychiatry* 75:518–524.
12. Scheib J., Riordan M., and Rubin S. 2005. Adolescents with open identity sperm donors: Reports from 12 to 17 years old. *Human Reprod* 20:239–252.

25

IUI and Psychological Aspects

Chris Verhaak and Jacky Boivin

From the start of reproductive treatments, attention has been paid to its emotional burden, which could be explained from the perspective of the treatment process as well as from the perspective of the unfulfilled child wish. It is generally recommended that a couple unsuccessfully trying to conceive for one year without prior reason for reduced fertility should be referred for further diagnostic testing, with subsequent treatment options likely to vary from expectant management to first-line interventions (e.g., insemination, ovulation induction) to IVF, ICSI, or even PESA or TESE (see e.g., NICE guidelines, ESHRE, ASRM policy). Intra-uterine insemination (IUI) consists of depositing via catheter partner or donor sperm into the intra-uterine cavity at the time of ovulation. Insemination can be accompanied by ovarian stimulation or only insemination within the natural cycle. IUI (with/without stimulation) is considered less invasive from a physical point of view because of the limited medical interventions involved, but, also from a psychological point of view because as a first-line treatment it means that if treatment fails other treatment options remain. The emotional burden of IVF and other assisted reproductive treatments (ART) is heightened by the last chance aspect of this treatment whereas the emotional burden of IUI is lessened by the possibility of an ART option as a next step in treatment.

This chapter describes the emotional aspects of IUI from the perspective of the threat of childlessness, psychological aspects of the treatment itself, the decision to start IUI, and the burden of different aspects of the treatment. The psychological aspects of expectant management or less invasive treatment before IVF or ICSI treatment is presented from the perspective of shared decision making.

The Burden of Subfertility: Multi-Dimensional Stressor

To understand the burden of IUI, it is important to have insight into the emotional impact of subfertility as such. Subfertility is a multi-dimensional source of stress. The emotional impact could be explained from the perspective of threat and loss. Threat is evoked by the treatment itself and the uncertainty of its outcome as well as by the prospective of a future life without children. Loss is evoked because of loss of the intimacy of conception, the loss of the experience of a spontaneous pregnancy, loss of dreams of a family, loss of possibility of giving grandchildren to your parents, and loss of feelings of relatedness with friends and family. Threat easily evokes anxiety (e.g., being tense, nervous, worried), while loss could result in a depressed mood (e.g., feeling sad, upset, disappointed). From the perspective of threat and loss, one would expect anxiety to be more apparent in IUI because loss could be postponed by the prospect of other treatment possibilities.

Emotional Health

Most studies into emotional health in subfertile couples are based on couples in IVF treatment or on subfertile couples in general (mostly only the women) irrespective of the type of treatment or phase in the treatment process. When studies do concern insemination, these are mainly comparing insemination with or without donor sperm, so that the donor aspect is the focus and not the insemination procedure per se. There is a lack of studies focusing on the emotional health of couples before, during, or after IUI.

The difference between couples going to start IUI versus those to start ART is that a considerable part of those in ART treatment already went through several less invasive treatments. Very few studies target patients in treatments before ART and those that do, do not differentiate between ovulation induction and assisted insemination versus IVF, ICSI, or even PESA or TESE.

Studies into emotional health in couples starting IVF show conflicting results. A review of studies investigating depression and anxiety before the start of IVF concluded that depression levels did not differ from norms whereas results on anxiety were equivocal: some studies showed no differences from norms, but a considerable number showed enhanced anxiety levels in women starting IVF. This supports the assumption that threat, and the uncertainty of outcome, is a more important driver of emotions during treatment than is the loss experienced from beliefs of impending permanent childlessness or an unfulfilled wish for a next child.

What is known from the emotional status in couples before they start ART, what could be understood as the transitional phase between IUI and ART, is that there does not seem to be a marked difference from norm groups on emotional distress. This suggests that unsuccessful IUI does not evoke high distress that continues in the starting period of the next treatment, which could be explained by the hope generated by the new treatment possibilities.

Adherence to Treatment

Despite favorable prognosis, a considerable group of women do not continue treatment even when there are remaining treatment options. Research shows that several types of reasons were indicated to explain discontinuation, but there are only a few studies taking reasons as well as phase in the process of fertility treatment into account.

Brandes and colleagues[3] carried out observational studies into the course of fertility treatment from first referral to specialized medical care until a year after the last treatment. In one study, they investigated the process of 1,391 couples through treatment. The treatment process was divided into six stages from first consult about fertility to advanced ART treatment. Specifically, couples that discontinued at stage 1 did not even start fertility work-up, stage 2 was during diagnostic fertility work-up, stage 3 was after work-up but before the start of fertility treatment, stage 4 was during or after ovulation induction or IUI but before ART, stage 5 was before third cycle IVF/ICSI, and stage 6 was after third cycle IVF/ICSI. Couples were followed up even when they moved to another clinic. The results showed that even before any treatment had started there was discontinuation with 144 out of 1,328 (11%, spontaneous pregnancies were excluded). During or after conventional treatment, it was another 9%. Data on reasons for discontinuation was provided for each stage of treatment, and these showed that reasons do differ according to this factor.

Figure 25.1 provides reason data in relation to the use of first-line treatments. Figure 25.1 indicates that during or after ovulation induction or IUI, the most frequently mentioned reason for discontinuation of treatment was emotional distress, whereas before conventional treatment, the most frequently mentioned reason was rejection of treatment in general. Rejection of treatment could indicate a desire not to medicalize the process of conception, erroneous beliefs (e.g., high chance of birth defects) or negative attitudes about treatment, an acceptance of infertility, or low need to resolve infertility (by treatment or otherwise). When couples started IVF or ICSI, the most frequent reason for discontinuation was poor prognosis and that is particularly true after a third unsuccessful treatment cycle, discontinuation

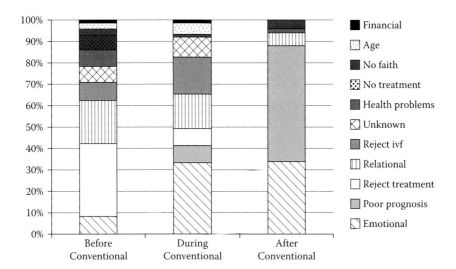

FIGURE 25.1   Percentage of reasons indicated for discontinuation of treatment by phase in treatment: before first-line treatment, during first-line treatment, or after first-line treatment.

before the third cycle is also frequently explained by emotional distress. These data argue against the assumption that less invasive or first-line treatments are not as burdensome as more invasive treatments like IVF.

Stress Induced by the Treatment

IUI imposes a larger burden if stimulation of follicles is involved. The physical discomfort of the treatment, together with logistic aspects concerning injections at fixed times, the need to attend a clinic for monitoring of follicle growth, and interaction with medical staff about progress of treatment could all contribute to this burden. We know from studies on emotional impact of ART that despite these important sources of stress, waiting for the pregnancy test is for most couples much more stressful than the other aspects of treatment. It is assumed that waiting for the pregnancy test after IUI would generate a similar pattern of emotional effects. Important differences, however, are the relatively short cycle of the treatment, one can start again soon, and, as noted, the prospect of other treatment possibilities in case of failure, which could all lessen emotional distress.

IUI: Time Delay or First Choice?

The best treatment option, especially for couples with unexplained fertility problems, is a frequent focus of discussion among clinicians. This is particularly true for the optimal number of IUIs that should be performed to achieve best chances of live birth. There is still a lack of consensus when IUI is recommended over IVF. Decisions are made on evidence about effect of different treatment options, but conclusive evidence is lacking in many situations. Further, patient preferences play a role in clinicians' decisions to opt for IVF against IUI. It sometimes seems difficult to convince couples that less invasive treatments such as IUI or even expectant management are the first choice of treatment in particular cases. Therefore, one of the emotionally stressful aspects of IUI for people could be due to the urge couples feel to move directly to IVF treatment, and the disappointment they experience when an alternative course of treatment is proposed. Research indicates that, even if there are evidence-based guidelines for differentiating between different types of ART, doctors have difficulties adhering to these guidelines when choosing treatment options with their patients. This inconsistency in medical

TABLE 25.1

Statements of Chapter 25

Statement	Level of Evidence (LOE)
Discontinuation during conventional fertility treatment or in between conventional treatment and ART is about 9%	3
Most important reasons for discontinuation of conventional fertility treatment are rejection of treatment and relational problems	3
Doctors have difficulties adhering to guidelines for conventional fertility treatment	3

TABLE 25.2

Recommendations of Chapter 25

Recommendation	Grade Strength
Adherence to guidelines for conventional fertility treatment and ART could alleviate uncertainty in patients	GPP
Clear information about reasons behind recommendation for conventional treatment will support patients' preference for this treatment option	D

policy could negatively affect patients because patients may become aware of it via discussion with other patients, information they get from other sources such as the Internet, divergence of recommendation between that received from different doctors in the same clinic, and so on. Since subfertility and its treatment are accompanied by much uncertainty for couples, limiting uncertainty from the part of the treatment team could reduce additional distress in couples, making them better able to follow recommendations for expectant management or first-line treatments instead of ART. This means that it is important to inform patients referred to specialized care that expectancy could be the more favorable option, above active treatment, or that IUI could be preferable above IVF. This is supported by Van den Boogaard et al.[1] showing that patients prefer to be informed about expectant management as one of the treatment options already early in the process, at their first visit to the clinic to better frame their expectations. The family practitioner too, could take this into account in counseling patients for reference to a specialized clinic.

Studies show that, for patients, characteristics of the treatment itself are not crucial in their preference for a specific treatment option. Couples seem to decide on perceived effectiveness of the treatment options. This means that in counseling couples for IUI, focus should be on success rates compared to other treatments rather than on factors related to convenience. On the other hand, if patients do not trust their doctor in recommendations for treatment, stress will increase and it will be much more difficult to deliberate pros and cons of different treatment options.

In conclusion, there is a lack of research on the emotional impact of IUI. We have to translate what is known from studies in allied patient groups to the situation of patients in IUI. If we do so we can conclude that IUI as a treatment seems to be not as stressful as ART because of the treatment options left. However, decisions about starting IUI instead of ART, or decisions about making the step from IUI to ART, put an additional burden on the treatment. Clinics can alleviate this burden from the very beginning by providing patients clear information about preferred treatment options in different situations. In addition, they should be aware of policies regarding treatment decisions in other clinics, and explain them to patients (see also Tables 25.1 and 25.2).

REFERENCES

1. Van den Boogaard N.M., Musters A.M., Brühl S.W., Tankens T., Kremer J.A., Mol B.W., Hompes P.G., Nelen W.L., and Van der Veen F. 2012. Tailored expectant management: A nationwide survey to quantify patients' and professionals' barriers and facilitators. *Hum Reprod* April 27(4):1050–7.

2. Boivin J., Domar A.D., Shapiro D.B., Wischmann T.H., Fauser B.C., Verhaak C. 2012. Tackling burden in ART: An integrated approach for medical staff. *Hum Reprod* April 27(4):941–50.
3. Brandes M., Van der Steen J.O., Bokdam S.B., Hamilton C.J., de Bruin J.P., Nelen W.L., and Kremer J.A. 2009. When and why do subfertile couples discontinue their fertility care? A longitudinal cohort study in a secondary care subfertility population. *Hum Reprod* December 24(12):3127–35.
4. Verhaak C.M., Smeenk J.M., Evers A.W., Kremer J.A., Kraaimaat F.W., and Braat D.D. 2007. Women's emotional adjustment to IVF: A systematic review of 25 years of research. *Hum Reprod Update* January–February 13(1):27–36.

26

Risk Factors for Higher-Order Multiple Pregnancies Following Stimulated IUI

Alexandra J. Bensdorp, Ben Willem Mol, and Fulco van der Veen

Introduction

Higher-Order Multiple Pregnancies (HOMPs) are defined as pregnancies with three or more fetuses. Higher-Order Multiple Births (HOMBs) are defined as deliveries of three or more babies. The frequency of HOMB after natural conception is described by Hellin's law; if twin births occur once in N births, then triplet births occur once in N^2 births and quadruplet births occur once in N^3 births.[1] Spontaneous twin births occur at a rate of 1 in 50 to 1 in 100 births (1 to 2%). Thus, spontaneous higher-order multiple births (HOMB) can be expected to occur in around 0.05% of all deliveries.

Over the last decades there has been a four- to eightfold increase in HOMBs, exceeding the numbers predicted by Hellin's law by far.[2,3] This explosive growth is mainly attributed to fertility treatments.[4] The sparse data in the literature suggests that non-IVF ovarian stimulation is responsible for 35–50% of all multiple pregnancies.[5-7] Unfortunately, data on an increase of the higher-order multiple births caused by intra-uterine insemination (IUI) with ovarian (hyper)stimulation (IUI/OH) are lacking, but it is estimated that ovarian hyperstimulation was responsible for 20% of twin births and for 38% of triplet and higher-order multiple births.[8]

At the European Society of Human Reproduction and Embryology consensus meeting in 2002, it was agreed that the preferred outcome of fertility treatment should be the birth of one healthy child, and that twin pregnancies, and thus also HOMPs, should be considered a complication.[9] Since then the number of multiple pregnancies after assisted reproductive technology (ART) has decreased as fewer embryos are being transferred. As no measures were undertaken to decrease the number of HOMBs following IUI their relative contribution increased between 1997 and 2000.[10]

IUI and the Incidence of Multiple Pregnancy

IUI is a common treatment for a broad range of subfertility diagnoses. Cumulative pregnancy rates with IUI/OH vary between 20 and 30% after six cycles, depending on the cause and duration of subfertility. In many countries IUI is more accessible than IVF or IVF/ICSI.

In 2007, 23 European countries reported 142,609 IUI cycles, where in 2001, 15 European countries reported 67,124 cycles of IUI.[11,12] In uncontrolled studies, pregnancy rates per cycle were 9.2%, but at the expense of considerable multiple pregnancy rates. Rates of twins and triplets were 11.4 and 0.6%, respectively, in 2005. Unfortunately, IUI data are not reported separately in the United States.

Potentially, the actual triplet conception rate following IUI is twice as high as reported, since 50% of triplet and higher-order pregnancies undergo spontaneous reduction to lower orders during the first trimester. In ongoing HOMPs, fetal reductions are often being performed thus reducing the numbers. To what extent the proportion of triplet deliveries would have been without these costly fetal reductions is unclear since national fetal reduction rates are not registered in national databases.

Maternal and Neonatal Risks of Higher-Order Multiple Pregnancies

Women carrying HOMP are at an increased risk of diabetes, pregnancy-induced hypertension, pre-eclampsia, and delivery through a caesarean section as well as postpartum hemorrhage. These risks are increased by an additional 20–50% in comparison to twin pregnancies, except for caesarean section, which approaches 100% in women delivering an HOMP. The largest cohort of triplets described a total of 198 women, and 94% were delivered by caesarean section.[13]

Neonatal complications associated with HOMPs are predominantly related to premature delivery (respiratory distress syndrome, bronchopulmonary dysplasia, intraventricular bleeding, and pneumonia). Recent U.S. data supplied by 426 fertility clinics show that after 138,198 cycles of IVF/ICSI, 95% of triplets or more compared to 63% of twins were born preterm. There is no reason to assume that HOMPs after IUI treatment would behave differently. The risk of a very preterm delivery (birth at <29 weeks of gestation) is increased for triplets and quadruplets compared with twins by a factor of 4 and 8, respectively.[14]

Growth restriction is another risk for children delivered from multiple pregnancies, and is increased by 42 to 57%. Low birth weight infants are more at risk for short and long-term disability such as cerebral palsy, mental retardation, and limited motor and cognitive skills. U.S. data show that low birth weight (<2500 gram) was found in 90% of the triplets and more, compared with 57% of the twins, and 8% of the singleton pregnancies. Mortality rates are six times higher for HOMPs when compared to singletons.[15]

Financial Consequences

Higher-order pregnancies are expensive; obstetric costs and perinatal costs are substantially higher than in singleton or twin pregnancies. Obstetrical costs include medication, as well as hospital admission and sometimes even emergency surgery. Obstetric costs are four to five times higher for triplets, and sevenfold for quadruplets compared to singletons.[16] Perinatal costs are enormous, and mostly associated with prematurity and dysmaturity.[17,18]

Admission costs to the neonatal intensive care unit are high and result in a two to fourfold increase in cost per child born. It has been estimated that the costs of an infant with extremely low birth weight, which is defined as <1000 g, vary between $45,000 and $60,000 depending on the country of treatment.[18] Additionally, the long-term costs due to handicaps like spastic cerebral palsy are substantial, and subsequently a burden for society.[16]

Risk Factors for HOMPs

In a recent meta-analysis of 14 studies with 11,599 IUI cycles, multi-follicular growth was associated with increased pregnancy rates in IUI with OH. Absolute pregnancy rates were 8.4% for mono-follicular growth, and 15% for multi-follicular growth. In cycles with three to four follicles, the multiple pregnancy rate increased without a substantial gain in overall pregnancy rate.[19]

In addition to the number of developing follicles, various authors have found a relation between multi-follicular growth, estradiol levels, female age, and HOMP rates. In 3,347 stimulated IUI cycles, the incidence of triplets and higher-order pregnancies was significantly related to the total number of follicles ≥7 mm and E2 concentration ≥1385 pg/mL (CHL assay).[20] The rate of HOMP was 3.8% if there were fewer than 15 follicles ≥7 mm and E2 concentration was below the earlier mentioned threshold. If there were more than 15 follicles ≥7 mm and E2 concentration was above the threshold, the HOMP rate reported was 22.2%.

In a prospective Spanish study, which aimed to build a prediction model for HOMP, these results were confirmed albeit with slightly different thresholds. In 1,542 stimulated IUI cycles, 2.4% of the pregnancies were triplet pregnancies. If the woman's age was below 32 years, and the E2 concentration was above the equivalent of 862 pg/mL (CHL assay) and the number of follicles ≥10 mm was more than five, women were considered a high-risk population. Of the pregnancies in this group, 6.9% were triplet, whereas for the low-risk group only 0.7% of the pregnancies was a triplet.[21]

Findings from the most recent study on this subject concur; for women of 38 years and older, no triplets and higher-order pregnancies occurred in 4,062 cycles of stimulated IUI. For the slightly younger women (33–37 years) the HOMP rate was 16.7%, and for the even younger ones (<32 yrs) the HOMP rate was 19.3% when there were seven or more follicles ≥10 mm present with an E2 concentration ≥ 1000 pg/ml by CHL. For the whole group, the incidence of HOMP was increased from 5 to 6% with four to six follicles present, to 14% with seven to eight follicles present, and to 19% with nine or more follicles present.[8]

As women are more prone to conceive in their first three treatment cycles, the risk for HOMP is especially high in these cycles. Four large retrospective studies show that practically no HOMP occurred after the third cycle.[8] More specifically, one study describes that HOMP did not occur after the first cycle unless there were more than seven follicles, and did not occur after the second cycle regardless of the number of follicles.[8]

Prevention of HOMPs

The first step to prevent HOMP is to evaluate whether fertility treatment is necessary in the first place. Patients for IUI/OH should be carefully selected. Prediction models can be used to do this. Chapter two elaborates on this subject.

As the number of follicles on the day of administering hCG is related to the number of HOMBs, only low dose stimulation protocols should be used. Already in 1970, no multiple pregnancies or HOMBs were found after a starting dosage of 75 IU HMG compared to a 13% twinning rate and 4.8% HOMB when stimulating with 150 IU of HMG.[22]

In a retrospective Italian study of 1,259 cycles with a low starting dose of 50 IU good pregnancy rates (15.8–21.9%) were obtained with 10% twins, without any higher-order pregnancies. Approximately 5% of cycles had to be canceled because of hyperresponse (predefined as three or more follicles ≥16 mm, and/or five or more follicles ≥ 11 mm).[23]

In a review including 10 studies that followed a low dose protocol, administering ≤75 IU FSH, clinical pregnancy rates per cycle varied from 9 to 20%, with a mean clinical pregnancy rate of 11% per cycle; triplets and higher-order pregnancy rates were kept to a minimum and varied between 0 and 2.4%. When cancellation criteria were applied in addition to the low dose protocol, the mean clinical pregnancy rate was 10% per cycle, and the HOMP frequency was further reduced to 0.3%.

If after careful selection of patients, and using low stimulation protocol patients are still at risk for HOMP, cancellation is the most frequently applied strategy in the prevention of HOMPs during IUI cycles. The American College of Obstetrics and Gynecology (ACOG) recommend canceling cycles or withholding hCG when more than three follicles are >15 mm and the Royal College of Obstetrics and Gynaecologists sets this threshold at >16 mm. Yet there is no consistent evidence to support either of these precautionary measures.

Instead of cancellation there are several other options for reducing the risk of a HOMP such as aspiration of supernumerary follicles, conversion to IVF, and multi-fetal pregnancy reduction. These options are described in the next chapter.

Summary and Conclusions

Triplets and higher-order pregnancies remain a major problem in IUI/OH. To prevent HOMP, prediction models can be used to distinguish patients with a good prognosis for a spontaneous pregnancy. In this patient group expectant management needs to be considered. With mild stimulation protocols and monitoring, particularly in young women and especially in their first cycles, most high-order multiples can be prevented. When primary prevention fails, canceling of cycles or aspiration of supernumerary follicles are a low impact option for secondary prevention (see also Tables 26.1 and 26.2).

TABLE 26.1

Statements of Chapter 26

Statement	Level of Evidence (LOE)
In stimulated IUI cycles with 3 to 4 follicles the multiple pregnancy rate increased without substantial gain in overall pregnancy rate	1a
Multi-follicular growth, woman's age and estradiol levels are risk factors for HOMP after stimulated IUI cycles	1b
HOMPs are more likely to occur in the first three treatment cycles	1c

TABLE 26.2

Recommendations of Chapter 26

Recommendation	Grade Strength
To prevent HOMP, prediction models can be used to select those patients with a good prognosis for a spontaneous pregnancy. Expectant management needs to be considered for this group	A
With mild stimulation protocols and monitoring most HOMPS can be prevented	A
When primary prevention fails, canceling IUI cycles or aspirating supernumary follicles are a low impact option for secondary prevention	A

REFERENCES

1. Fellman J. and Eriksson A.W. 2009. Statistical analyses of Hellin's law. *Twin Res Hum Genet* 12:191–200.
2. Martin J.A. and Park M.M. 1999. Trends in twin and triplet births: 1980–97. *Natl Vital Stat Rep* 47:1–16.
3. Blickstein I. and Keith L.G. 2003. Outcome of triplets and high-order multiple pregnancies. *Curr Opin Obstet Gynecol* 15:113–117.
4. Keith L. and Oleszczuk J.J. 1999. Iatrogenic multiple birth, multiple pregnancy and assisted reproductive technologies. *Int J Gynaecol Obstet* 64:11–25.
5. Levene M.I., Wild J., and Steer P. 1992. Higher multiple births and the modern management of infertility in Britain. The British Association of Perinatal Medicine. *Br J Obstet Gynaecol* 99:607–613.
6. Bergh T., Ericson A., Hillensjo T., Nygren K.G., and Wennerholm U.B. 1999. Deliveries and children born after *in vitro* fertilisation in Sweden 1982–95: A retrospective cohort study. *Lancet* 354:1579–1585.
7. Tur R., Barri P.N., Coroleu B., Buxaderas R., Martinez F., and Balasch J. 2001. Risk factors for high-order multiple implantation after ovarian stimulation with gonadotrophins: Evidence from a large series of 1878 consecutive pregnancies in a single centre. *Hum Reprod* 16:2124–2129.
8. Dickey R.P., Taylor S.N., Lu P.Y., Sartor B.M., Rye P.H., and Pyrzak R. 2005. Risk factors for high-order multiple pregnancy and multiple birth after controlled ovarian hyperstimulation: Results of 4,062 intra-uterine insemination cycles. *Fertil Steril* 83:671–683.
9. Land J.A. and Evers J.L. 2003. Risks and complications in assisted reproduction techniques: Report of an ESHRE consensus meeting. *Hum Reprod* 18:455–457.
10. Reynolds M.A., Schieve L.A., Martin J.A., Jeng G., and Macaluso M. 2003. Trends in multiple births conceived using assisted reproductive technology, United States 1997–2000. *Pediatrics* May: 111 (5 Part 2):1159–1162.
11. Andersen A.N., Gianaroli L., Felberbaum R., deMouzon J., and Nygren K.G., European IVF-monitoring programme (EIM), European Society of Human Reproduction and Embryology (ESHRE). 2005. Assisted reproductive technology in Europe, 2001. Results generated from European registers by ESHRE. *Hum Reprod.* May 20(5):1158–76. Epub 2005, January 21.
12. de Mouzon J., Goossens V., Bhattacharya S., Castilla J.A, Ferraretti A.P., Korsak V., Kupka M., Nygren K.G., and Andersen A.N., European IVF-Monitoring (EIM), Consortium for the European Society on Human Reproduction and Embryology (ESHRE). 2012. Assisted reproductive technology in Europe, 2007: Results generated from European registers by ESHRE. *Hum Reprod* 27(4):954–966.
13. Newman R.B., Hamer C., and Miller M.C. 1989. Outpatient triplet management: A contemporary review. *Am J Obstet Gynecol* 161:547–553.

14. Luke B. and Brown M.B. 2008. Maternal morbidity and infant death in twin vs. triplet and quadruplet pregnancies. *Am J Obstet Gynecol* 198:401–410.
15. Alexander G.R., Slay W.M., Salihu H., and Kirby R.S. 2005. Fetal and neonatal mortality risks of multiple births. *Obstet Gynecol Clin North Am* 32:1–16, vii.
16. Mugford M. 1995. The cost of neonatal care: Reviewing the evidence. *Soz Praventiv Med* 40: 361–368.
17. Petrou S. and Henderson J. 2003. Preference-based approaches to measuring the benefits of perinatal care. *Birth* 30:217–226.
18. Ombelet W., De S.P., Van der Elst J., and Martens G. 2005. Multiple gestation and infertility treatment: Registration, reflection and reaction—The Belgian project. *Hum Reprod Update* 11:3–14.
19. Van Rumste M.M., Custers I.M., van der Veen F., van Wely M., Evers J.L., and Mol B.W. 2008. The influence of the number of follicles on pregnancy rates in intrauterine insemination with ovarian stimulation: A meta-analysis. *Hum Reprod Update* 14:563–570.
20. Gleicher N., Oleske D.M., Tur-Kaspa I., Vidali A., and Karande V. 2000. Reducing the risk of high-order multiple pregnancy after ovarian stimulation with gonadotrophins. *N Engl J Med* 343:2–7.
21. Tur R., Barri P., Coroleu B., Buxaderas R., Parera N., and Balasch J. 2005. Use of a prediction model for high-order multiple implantation after ovarian stimulation with gonadotrophins. *Fertil Steril* 83(1):116–121.
22. Thompson C.R. and Hansen L.M. 1970. Pergonal (menotropins): A summary of clinical experience in the induction of ovulation and pregnancy. *Fertil Steril* 21:844–853.
23. Ragni G., Caliari I., Nicolosi A.E., Arnoldi M., Somigliana E., and Crosignani P.G. 2006. Preventing high-order multiple pregnancies during controlled ovarian hyperstimulation and intrauterine insemination: 3 years' experience using low-dose recombinant follicle-stimulating hormone and gonadotropin-releasing hormone antagonists. *Fertil Steril* 85:619–624.

27

Prevention of Multiple Pregnancies after IUI

Diane de Neubourg, Jan Bosteels, and Thomas D'Hooghe

Introduction

Multiple pregnancies and high-order multiple pregnancies in particular are an undesired side effect of any infertility treatment. However, the burden of the treatment itself or of an unfulfilled pregnancy should be taken into account when the couple is counseled about the possibilities to achieve a pregnancy. Intra-uterine insemination (IUI) is proposed in the case of mild male infertility, unexplained infertility, in the presence of mild endometriosis, or for cervical infertility. Although IUI is generally perceived as a low burden and low-risk therapy, the European IVF Monitoring[1] reported 11.7% twin deliveries and 0.5% triplets in 2007 in women <40 years treated with IUI using their husband's sperm. In 2005, ovarian hyperstimulation (OH) with IUI and ovarian hyperstimulation alone contributed as much as 22.8% to the national multiple birth cohort in the United States.[2]

In women treated by IUI, not only the pregnancy rate but also the risk of achieving a (high-order) multiple pregnancy is associated with the addition of OH and with the ovarian response to OH. Therefore, appropriate OH should be a balance between these two outcome variables, with a focus on the complete prevention of higher-order multiple pregnancies, and to reduce the twin pregnancies to the lowest possible rate.

Identification of Risk Factors

Prevention of multiple pregnancies should take into account the risk factors for multiple pregnancies, most importantly the number of follicles at the time of ovulation triggering, as discussed in the previous chapter. Assuming a 60% fertilization rate, as generally observed in ART programs, it appears logical to aim at more than one follicle during treatment with OH and IUI. A meta-analysis performed by Van Rumste et al. in 2008[3] included 14 studies reporting on 11,599 cycles; only two studies were randomized controlled trials in contrast to 12 observational studies. The absolute pregnancy rate was 8.4% for mono-follicular and 15% for multi-follicular growth. The pooled odds ratio (OR) for pregnancy after two follicles as compared with mono-follicular growth was 1.6 (99% confidence interval [CI] 1.3–2.0), whereas for three and four follicles, the pooled OR was 2.0 (99% CI 1.6–2.5) and 2.0 (95% CI 1.5–2.7), respectively. Compared with mono-follicular growth, pregnancy rates increased by 5, 8, and 8% when stimulating two, three, and four follicles, respectively. The pooled OR for multiple pregnancies after two follicles was 1.7 (99% CI 0.8–3.6), and increased to 2.8 and 2.3 for three and four follicles, respectively. The risk of multiple pregnancies after two, three, and four follicles increased by 6, 14, and 10%. The absolute rate of multiple pregnancies was 0.3% after mono-follicular and 2.8% after multi-follicular growth. It was concluded that multi-follicular growth is associated with increased pregnancy rates in IUI with OH.[3] Treatment combining OH and IUI should not aim for more than two follicles, since in cycles with three or four follicles the multiple pregnancy rate increased without substantial gain in overall pregnancy rate. One stimulated follicle should be the goal if prevention of multiple pregnancies is the primary concern, whereas two follicles may be acceptable after careful patient counseling (see also Tables 27.1 and 27.2).

Analysis of the Risks of Different Stimulation Protocols for Multiple Pregnancies

In a narrative review, McClamrock et al.[2] compared the reproductive outcome after OH with clomiphene citrate, low-dose gonadotrophins (≤75 IU), and high-dose gonadotrophins (≥150 IU) in combination with IUI (see Table 27.3). They retrieved data from randomized controlled trials on the different stimulation protocols, analyzed them accordingly, but without formal meta-analysis. The authors[2] concluded first that an increasingly compelling case can be made in support of low-dose (≤75 IU) gonadotrophin regimens, for which per-cycle pregnancy rates of 8.7–16.3% and absent high-order gestation have been noted in prospective randomized trials, although a more mixed record was noted for the twin gestation category. A second conclusion[2] was that a strong case can also be made for clomiphene for which per-cycle pregnancy rates of 2.0–19.3% have been noted in prospective, randomized trials, with virtual absence of high-order gestation, and twin gestation rates ranging between 0 and 12.5%. However, these conclusions should be interpreted cautiously since they are based on a nonsystematic narrative review of the literature[2] without accounting for many forms of bias.

In a more thorough systematic *Cochrane Review*[4] on the influence of the type of ovarian stimulation combined with IUI, it was concluded that OH using gonadotrophins increases the pregnancy rates compared with the use of anti-estrogens (OR = 1.8, 95% CI 1.2 to 1.7). For the studies that could be included in the comparison,[4] there appeared to be no difference in the multiple pregnancy rate after OH with gonadotrophins or anti-estrogens when calculated per patient (OR = 0.53, 95% CI 0.15–1.86) or per pregnancy (OR = 0.96, 95% CI 0.28–3.28). Doubling the starting dose of gonadotrophins did not increase pregnancy rates (OR = 1.2, 95% CI 0.67 to 1.9) or affect multiple pregnancy rates (OR = 3.11, 95% CI 0.48–20.13). Based on this systematic review, OH with gonadotrophins is superior to OH with anti-estrogens in an IUI program, without concomitant increased risk in multiple pregnancy rate. Nevertheless, it should be kept in mind that the risk for multiple pregnancy rates is more dependent on the number of stimulated follicles than on the type of product used for OH (gonadotrophins or clomiphene citrate), as reviewed above in the section "Identification of Risk Factors."

To further optimize the dosage of gonadotrophins in gonadotrophin-stimulated insemination cycles, a study was performed by la Cour Freiesleben et al.,[5] who developed and pilot tested a tailored stimulation schedule for a recombinant follicle-stimulating hormone (rFSH) dosage nomogram. In a multi-center randomized controlled trial, 228 ovulatory patients scheduled for OH and IUI were randomized to *individual* (50–100 IU rFSH/day, n = 113) or *standard* (75 IU rFSH/day, n = 115) dose. Individual dose was prescribed according to the nomogram, which was based on patients' body weight and antral follicle count. The primary end point was the proportion of patients with two to three follicles ≥14 mm (maximum two follicles ≥18 mm) on the day of hCG (leading follicle = 18 mm). In the individual group, 79/113 (70%) of the patients developed two to three follicles versus 64/115 (56%) in the standard

TABLE 27.3

Pregnancy and Multiple Pregnancy Rate with Clomiphene Citrate and Gonadotrophins Combined with IUI, According to Narrative Review

	Number of Cycles	Pregnancy Rate per Cycle (%)	Twin Intra-Uterine Pregnancy Rate (%)	High-Order Intra-Uterine Pregnancy Rate (%)
Clomiphene citrate	3214	2–19.3	0–12.5	0–3.7
Low dose gonadotrophins (≤75 IU)	1123	8.7–16.3	0–29.3	0
High dose gonadotrophins (≥150 IU)	2227	8.7–19.2	0–28.6	0–9.3

Source: McClamrock et al., 2012, *Fertil Steril* 4:802–9.

group (risk difference = 14%, 95% CI 2 to 26%, P = 0.03). Among patients with two to three follicles, the proportion of patients with two follicles was similar in the individual group (58%, 46/79) and in the standard group (53%; 34/64; P = 0.54). Individual and standard groups were also comparable with respect to ongoing pregnancy rates (20%; 23/113 versus 18%; 21/115) and multiple gestation rates (1%; 1/113 versus 4%; 5/115, P = 0.21). The authors[5] concluded that dosing according to the nomogram was superior to standard dosing. However, on the basis of the published results there is no evidence at present for a better benefit versus risk ratio using the doses according to the nomogram versus standard dosing. Probably the study[5] was underpowered and therefore more studies are needed to clarify this knowledge gap.

Secondary Preventive Measures

Cancellation of the Cycle

When multi-follicular development occurs during OH, a risk for (high-order) multiple pregnancies exists. As mentioned previously, on the basis of risk analysis by Van Rumste et al.,[3] one should aim for a maximum of two follicles in order to avoid high-order multiple pregnancies. Apart from common sense, there are no studies available where risks of the number of follicles and their size are weighed and evaluated. There is a lack of evidence-based guidelines. In Europe, only four of 25 countries have issued IUI guidelines considered of sufficient quality for use in daily practice.[6]

Aspiration of Supernumerary Follicles

Instead of cancellation of the cycle, supernumerary follicles can be aspirated vaginally under ultrasound guidance. In the studies reported, follicular aspiration was performed on the day of hCG administration when four or more follicles ≥ 14 mm were present. Three studies reported pregnancy rates and multiple pregnancy rates of 25–27% and 0–10%, respectively.[2] In our IUI program, routinely using selective aspiration of supernumerary follicles if three or more follicles sized 15 mm or more are present at the time of hCG administration, the live birth rate per cycle is 19–20%, whereas the multiple live birth rate per total number of pregnancies is about 4–6%.[7] Although these results suggest that selective follicular aspiration works in "real life" clinical practice, patients should be counseled about this "invasive" option before they start with an IUI program.

Escape IVF

When many follicles have to be aspirated, it is important to discuss the possibility of a full oocyte aspiration performed as part of an ART treatment. This rescue procedure can certainly increase the chance of achieving a pregnancy with minimal risks for multiple pregnancies, provided single embryo transfer is performed. However, the costs associated with ART are much higher than those associated with IUI. Furthermore, success of ART treatment can be compromised if oocytes ovulate prematurely, a common problem as most patients are not treated with a GnRH analogue or antagonist in the context of OH and IUI. In principle, GnRH antagonist can be added during OH, but this is not always possible since follicle size usually exceeds 14 mm at the time of the decision to switch from IUI to IVF.

Selective Reduction of a Multi-Fetal Pregnancy

High-order multiple pregnancies will be at increased risk for adverse maternal and perinatal outcome. The balance between reducing the number of fetuses in an attempt to decrease maternal and perinatal risks versus continuation of the pregnancy has to be made individually based on patient counseling provided by ultrasound interventionalists, subspecialists in fetal–maternal medicine, neonatologists, and psychologists.

TABLE 27.1

Statements of Chapter 27

Statement	Level of Evidence (LOE)
Pregnancy is more likely to occur with two follicles than with one[a]	1a
The risk of multiple pregnancies for two follicles as compared to mono-follicular growth increases by 6%[a]	1a
Higher pregnancy rates are obtained in IUI when combined with gonadotrophins compared to anti-estrogen[b]	1a
Doubling the dose of gonadotrophins does not increase the pregnancy rate[b]	1a

[a] From Van Rumste et al., 2008, *Hum Reprod Update* 6:563–70.
[b] From Cantineau and Cohlen, 2011, *Cochrane Database Syst Rev* 6:CD005356.

TABLE 27.2

Recommendations of Chapter 27

Recommendation	Grade Strength
When combined with IUI, low dose gonadotrophins should be used instead of high dose gonadotrophins[a]	A
IUI combined with gonadotrophin treatment adjusted by nomogram is superior to standard dosing of 75 IU[b]	B
OH with IUI should aim for no more than two follicles[c]	A
Follicle aspiration can prevent multiple pregnancies while maintaining acceptable pregnancy rates[d,e]	B or C
In case of multi-follicular development, escape ART (conversion from IUI into ART) can prevent multiple pregnancies while maintaining acceptable pregnancy rates, when combined with single embryo transfer[d]	B or C

[a] From Cantineau and Cohlen, 2011, *Cochrane Database Syst Rev* 6:CD005356.
[b] From la Cour Freiesleben et al., 2009, *Hum Reprod* 24:2523–30.
[c] From Van Rumste et al., 2008, *Hum Reprod Update* 6:563–70.
[d] From McClamrock et al., 2012, *Fertil Steril* 4:802–9.
[e] ESHRE, 2009, *Hum Reprod Update* 3:265–77.

REFERENCES

1. de Mouzon J., Goossens V., Bhattacharya S., Castilla J.A., Ferraretti A.P., Korsak V., Kupka M., Nygren K.G., Andersen A.N., and European IVF-Monitoring (EIM), Consortium for the European Society on Human Reproduction and Embryology (ESHRE). 2012. Assisted reproductive technology in Europe, 2007: Results generated from European registers by ESHRE. *Hum Reprod* 24:954–66.
2. McClamrock H.D., Jones H.W. Jr., and Adashi E.Y. 2012. Ovarian stimulation and intra-uterine insemination at the quarter centennial: Implications for the multiple births epidemic. *Fertil Steril* 4:802–9.
3. Van Rumste M.M., Custers I.M., Van der Veen F., Van Wely M., Evers J.L., and Mol B.W. 2008. The influence of the number of follicles on pregnancy rates in intra-uterine insemination with ovarian stimulation: A meta-analysis. *Hum Reprod Update* 6:563–70.
4. Cantineau A.E. and Cohlen B.J. 2011. Ovarian stimulation protocols (anti-oestrogens, gonadotrophins with and without agonists/antagonists) for intra-uterine insemination (IUI) in women with subfertility. *Cochrane Database Syst Rev* 6:CD005356.
5. la Cour Freiesleben N., Lossl K., Bogstad J., Bredkjaer H.E., Toft B., Rosendahl M., Loft A., Bangsboll S., Pinborg A., and Nyboe Andersen A. 2009. Individual versus standard dose of rFSH in a mild stimulation protocol for intra-uterine insemination: A randomized study. *Hum Reprod* 24:2523–30.
6. ESHRE Capri Workshop Group. 2009. Intra-uterine insemination. *Hum Reprod Update* 3:265–77.
7. Vermeylen A.M., D'Hooghe T., Debrock S., Meeuwis L., Meuleman C., and Spiessens C. 2006. The type of catheter has no impact on the pregnancy rate after intra-uterine insemination: A randomized study. *Hum Reprod* 21:2364–7.

28

Perinatal Outcome after IUI

Willem Ombelet and Petra de Sutter

Introduction

Intra-uterine insemination (IUI), with or without ovarian stimulation, is a widely used treatment option for many subfertile couples in case of unexplained infertility, mild endometriosis, and mild or moderate male subfertility. Because IUI is a cost-effective and less invasive first-line treatment compared to IVF, it is nowadays the most frequently used treatment option of assisted reproduction worldwide.

It was shown before that the perinatal outcome of pregnancies caused by assisted reproductive technology (ART) is substantially worse when compared to pregnancies following natural conception (NC).[1] This is mainly attributed to a higher rate of multiple births, which in turn is associated with a higher rate of perinatal mortality and morbidity. In ovarian hyperstimulation (OH), the prediction of multiple gestation is highly uncertain especially when gonadotrophins are used. Because of the widespread use of gonadotrophins, induction of ovulation (OI), and OH, with or without artificial insemination, have become the main cause of multiple pregnancies related to infertility treatment in the United States. The outcome of births reported to the Centers for Disease Control for IVF for the years 2000–2003 showed that IVF accounts for about 8% of twin births, OI/COH for about 30%, and natural twinning for the remainder. For triplets, IVF accounts for 15%, OI/OE 65%, and natural twinning for the residual 20%.[2]

However, even for singleton pregnancies it has been shown that the outcome is worse after IVF/ICSI as compared to spontaneous pregnancies. This has been attributed to various factors, but mainly the treatment technology itself and/or the underlying infertility problem of the couple.

Very few studies have investigated the perinatal outcome following IUI. An important question is whether pregnancy and neonatal outcome is also worse following AI in singleton pregnancies, as it is for IVF pregnancies, compared to spontaneous pregnancies. In this respect, De Sutter et al.[3] have shown that there was no difference in the outcome of IUI versus IVF pregnancies in a matched case-control study of twice 126 patients. Since IVF is a much more artificial technique than IUI, the conclusion of that study was that the worse outcome of singleton pregnancies following ART was not due to the techniques of ART but to the infertility itself.

Methods/Results

To our knowledge only four papers have been published reporting the obstetric and perinatal outcome after IUI in a direct comparison with spontaneous conceptions, with contradictory results. According to Nuojua-Huttunen et al.[4] and using the data obtained from the Finnish Medical Birth Register (MBR), IUI treatment did not increase obstetric or perinatal risks compared with matched spontaneous or, more surprisingly, IVF pregnancies. In this study, 111 IUI pregnancies were compared with 333 spontaneous and 333 IVF pregnancies. Wang et al.[5] examined preterm birth in 1,015 IUI/AID singleton births compared to 1,019 IVF/ICSI and 1,019 NC births. They found that singleton IUI/AID births were about 1.5 times more likely to be born preterm than NC singletons, whereas the IVF/ICSI group were 2.4 times more likely to be born preterm than the NC group. They found no significant difference in the risk of preterm birth for IUI (partner semen) compared to DI (donor semen) within their *low technology* group (7.0% versus 7.5%, respectively).

In a retrospective cohort study, Gaudoin et al.[6] described a poorer perinatal outcome of singletons born to subfertile mothers conceived through OHIUI compared to matched natural conceptions within the Scottish national cohort, comparing 133 OH/AI pregnancies with 109,443 pregnancies of the Scottish national cohort. This difference in perinatal outcome was caused by a higher incidence of prematurity and low-birth-weight infants. They concluded that the perinatal outcome of singletons after OH/AI is poorer and associated with low birth weight, but only when IUI was done with partner's semen and not with donor semen.

The largest study to date[7] was performed in Flanders investigating differences in perinatal outcome of singleton and twin pregnancies after OH, with or without artificial insemination, compared to pregnancies after natural conception. Data were obtained from the Study Centre for Perinatal Epidemiology of Flanders (SPE). The outcome of 661,065 births could be investigated: 11,938 singleton and 3,108 twin births. Control NC subjects were matched for maternal age, parity, fetal sex, plurality, place, and year of birth. A significantly higher incidence of extreme prematurity (<32 weeks), very low birth weight (<1500 grams), stillbirths, and perinatal death for OH/AI singletons could be observed (Table 28.3). Twin pregnancies resulting from OH/AI showed a higher rate of neonatal mortality, assisted ventilation and respiratory distress syndrome when compared to NC pregnancies. Because mono-chorionicity is highly associated with an increased perinatal mortality and morbidity, the authors also studied the data of unlike-sex twins only. In this selected group of dizygotic pregnancies (42.5% of all twin pregnancies after OH/AI treatment in this study) they observed a significantly higher rate of very low birth weight and extreme prematurity for the OH/AI group compared to the NC comparison group (Table 28.4).

Discussion

The reason why perinatal health problems occur more frequently in non-IVF pregnancies compared to natural conception is still unknown, but can be explained by the procedure itself (IUI), the endocrine changes caused by ovarian stimulation medication, or the reason for infertility as such. Because the increased risk for multiple pregnancies after non-IVF hormonal treatment is comparable with IVF/ICSI, especially when gonadotrophins are used, this may also be an important factor influencing the worse perinatal outcome of non-IVF singleton and twin pregnancies after OH/IUI.

TABLE 28.3

Comparison of Obstetric and Perinatal Data of 12,021 COS/AI and 12,021 Spontaneously Conceived Singleton Births, Matched for Parity, Maternal Age, Date of Birth, and Fetal Sex

Births	OH/IUI N = 12.021		Controls N = 12.021				
Perinatal data	N	%	N	%	OR (95% CI)	P-value	RR (95% CI)
GA<32 weeks	152	1.3	47	0.4	3.26 (2.32–4.59)	<0.001*	3.23 (2.33–4.48)
GA<37 weeks	938	7.8	514	4.2	1.89 (1.69–2.12)	<0.001*	1.28 (1.64–2.03)
Birth weight <1500 g	159	1.3	50	0.4	3.21 (2.31–4.47)	<0.001*	3.18 (2.31–4.26)
Birth weight <2500 g	794	6.6	441	3.7	1.86 (1.65–2.10)	<0.001*	1.80 (1.61–2.02)
Transfer to NICU	2194	18.3	1536	12.8	1.52 (1.42–1.64)	<0.001*	1.43 (1.35–1.52)
Perinatal death	91	0.76	70	0.58	1.30 (0.94–1.80)	0.11	1.30 (0.95–1.77)
Stillbirth	59	0.49	45	0.37	1.31 (0.88–1.97)	0.20	1.31 (0.89–1.93)
Neonatal death	32	0.27	25	0.21	1.28 (0.74–2.23)	0.42	1.28 (0.76–2.16)
Assisted ventilation	183	1.5	85	0.7	2.17 (1.66–2.84)	<0.001*	2.15 (1.67–2.78)
IC bleeding	46	0.4	14	0.1	3.29 (1.76–6.28)	<0.001*	3.28 (1.81–5.97)
RDS	102	0.8	40	0.3	2.56 (1.75–3.76)	<0.001*	2.55 (1.77–3.67)

Note: GA = gestational age, NICU = neonatal intensive care unit, IC = Intracranial, RDS = Respiratory Distress Syndrome.
* Statistically significant.

TABLE 28.4

Comparison of Obstetric and Perinatal Data of 1320 COS/AI and 1320 Spontaneously Conceived Unlike-Sex Twin Births, Matched for Parity, Maternal Age, Date of Birth, and Fetal Sex

Births	OH/IUI N = 1,320		Controls N = 1,320				
Perinatal data	N	%	N	%	OR (95% CI)	P-value	RR (95%CI)
GA < 32 weeks	114	8.6	85	6.4	1.37 (1.02–1.86)	0.033*	1.34 (1.02–1.76)
GA < 37 weeks	719	54.5	615	46.6	1.96 (1.67–2.31)	<0.001*	1.17 (1.08–1.26)
Birth weight <1500 g	119	9.0	90	6.8	1.61 (1.21–2.14)	0.037*	1.32 (1.02–1.72)
Birth weight <2500 g	764	57.8	669	50.7	1.14 (1.34–1.56)	<0.001*	1.14 (1.06–1.23)
Transfer to NICU	894	67.7	885	67.0	1.03 (0.87–1.22)	0.71	1.01 (0.96–1.07)
Perinatal death	45	3.41	29	2.19	1.57 (0.96–2.59)	0.06	1.55 (0.98–2.46)
Stillbirth	21	1.59	12	0.90	1.76 (0.82–3.82)	0.11	1.75 (0.86–3.54)
Neonatal death	24	1.85	17	1.28	1.42 (0.73–2.77)	0.26	1.41 (0.76–2.62)
Assisted ventilation	98	7.4	93	7.0	1.06 (0.78–1.44)	0.71	1.05 (0.80–1.38)
IC bleeding	25	1.9	26	1.9	1.04 (0.58–1.87)	0.89	0.96 (0.56–1.66)
RDS	82	6.2	73	5.5	1.13 (0.81–1.59)	0.46	1.12 (0.83–1.53)

Note: GA = gestational age, NICU = neonatal intensive care unit, IC = Intracranial, RDS = Respiratory Distress Syndrome.
* Statistically significant.

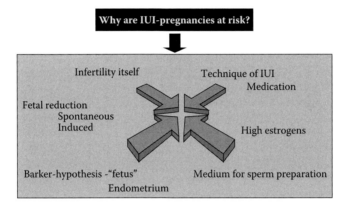

FIGURE 28.1   Factors that might be associated with an increased perinatal risk for IUI pregnancies.

It also seems that spontaneous reduction of multiple pregnancies causes a higher risk for adverse obstetric and perinatal outcome compared to pregnancies without spontaneous reduction. Indeed, it has been shown that the increased incidence of premature birth reported for IVF singleton and twin births, compared to NC pregnancies, is due in large part to the initial occurrence of triplet and higher-order gestations which will undergo spontaneous reduction in almost 50% of cases. These pregnancies continue as viable singleton and twin pregnancies, but they are at increased risk for prematurity compared to IVF singletons and twins that began as a singleton or twin gestation. More than 10% of IVF/ICSI singletons are the result of a vanishing twin, the same can be expected after IUI if gonadotrophins are used. Survivors of a vanishing cotwin have a higher risk for prematurity and low birth weight compared to singletons from single gestations.[8] Since we may expect that the rate of spontaneous reduction is comparable for IVF and non-IVF assisted reproductive techniques, this phenomenon can explain, at least partly, the worse perinatal health outcome after OH/IUI compared to natural conception singleton and twin pregnancies (Figure 28.1).

Considering singletons, it is not possible from the present study to tease out which potential causal factor (insemination procedure, medication used, the influence of vanishing twins, or the underlying infertility as such) is responsible for the difference in perinatal outcome between both groups. It, however, seems that the pregnancy and perinatal outcome is worse in the function of the severity of the infertility or the intensity of the treatment. In this respect, AI scores somewhere in the middle between spontaneous conceptions and IVF/ICSI.

Prevention of multiple pregnancies remains the cornerstone of success in non-IVF procedures using OH. When three or more follicles of a diameter greater than or equal to 15 mm are present, reasonable options are (a) to cancel the insemination procedure, (b) to prevent timed coitus during the following days, (c) to perform rescue IVF with or without the use of a GnRH antagonist, and/or (d) to do follicular aspiration. Trials with low dosage gonadotrophin protocols resulted in a lower multiple birth rate without influencing the ongoing pregnancy rate significantly. Clomiphene citrate (CC) remains a good first-line option with successful ovulation induction in about 50–70% of cases and a reasonable multiple pregnancy rate below 10%. Artificial insemination can be done in natural cycles, especially in case of cervical factor infertility, moderate male factor, and use of donor semen.

Artificial Insemination with Homologous Sperm (AIH) versus Artificial Insemination with Donor Sperm (AID)

Pregnancies resulting from donor insemination carry no increased risk compared to spontaneous gestations.[5,6,9] In a large French population study it was shown that after AID the miscarriage and tubal pregnancy rate, the children's weight, and the prematurity rate was not different from that of the general French population.[10] The birth chromosomal abnormalities rate is normal and correlated not only to the mother's age but also to the donor's age. As far as birth defects or chromosomal abnormalities are concerned, no difference has been observed from the general population. The use of frozen spermatozoa does not seem to affect the health of children conceived by AID. In other words, pregnancy outcome is not changed after sperm cryopreservation. On the other hand, IUI with donor sperm appears to increase the incidence of preeclampsia when pregnancy is achieved. A protective effect of multiple cycles also appears to be present in this respect.

Conclusions

According to the literature, OH/IUI singleton and twin pregnancies are significantly disadvantaged compared to naturally conceived children with a higher mortality rate and a higher incidence of low birth weight and prematurity. According to the results of this review we need to inform couples undergoing treatment with ovarian stimulation, with or without artificial insemination, about the increased risk of perinatal mortality and morbidity in twins compared to singletons. Low-dose protocols of ovarian stimulation are mandatory for the prevention of multiple pregnancies in artificial insemination. Couples should also be informed about an increased risk for perinatal health problems if they become pregnant after homologous IUI when compared to spontaneous pregnancies, even for singletons. A close follow-up of IUI pregnancies from the beginning is mandatory to detect spontaneous reduction of multiple pregnancies, which might be very important for that particular pregnancy. A pregnancy following artificial insemination has to be treated as a risk pregnancy (see also Tables 28.1 and 28.2).

TABLE 28.1

Statements of Chapter 28

Statement	Level of Evidence (LOE)
Singleton and twin pregnancies after IUI have a higher incidence of low birth weight, prematurity, and perinatal mortality and morbidity compared to natural conception pregnancies	2a
Multiple pregnancies are the most important factor affecting the perinatal outcome after IUI	2a
The addition of ovarian hyperstimulation requires a strict follow-up of the IUI cycle to prevent multiple pregnancies	2a

TABLE 28.2

Recommendations of Chapter 28

Recommendation	Grade Strength
When twins are to be prevented because of a higher perinatal morbidity and mortality, mono-follicular growth should be the aim	A
Preventive measures should be adapted if three or more follicles with a mean diameter of 14 mm or more are observed before ovulation/insemination	A
Couples should also be informed about an increased risk for perinatal health problems if they become pregnant after IUI	B
A pregnancy following artificial insemination has to be treated as a risk pregnancy	B

We need more research on the effect of ovarian stimulation on birth weight and perinatal outcome. In this respect it would be interesting to compare the perinatal outcome of IUI babies born after natural conception and IUI versus babies born after ovarian hyperstimulation and IUI.

REFERENCES

1. Helmerhorst F.M., Perquin D.A., Donker D., and Keirse M.J. 2004. Perinatal outcome of singletons and twins after assisted conception: A systematic review of controlled studies. *Brit Med J* 328:261–265.
2. Jones H.W. 2007. Iatrogenic multiple births: A 2003 checkup. *Fertil Steril* 87:453–455.
3. De Sutter P., Veldeman L., Kok P., Szymczak N., Van der Elst J., and Dhont M. 2005. Comparison of outcome of pregnancy after intra-uterine insemination (IUI) and IVF. *Hum Reprod* 20:1642–1646.
4. Nuojua-Huttunen S., Gissler M., Martikainen H., and Tuomivaara L. 1999. Obstetric and perinatal outcome of pregnancies after intra-uterine insemination. *Hum Reprod* 14:2110–2115.
5. Wang J.X., Norman R.J., and Kristiansson P. 2002. The effect of various infertility treatments on the risk of preterm birth. *Hum Reprod* 17:945–949.
6. Gaudoin M., Dobbie R., Finlayson A. et al. 2003. Ovulation induction/intra-uterine insemination in infertile couples is associated with low-birth-weight infants. *Am J Obstet Gynecol* 188:611–616.
7. Ombelet W., Martens G., DeSutter P. et al. 2006. Perinatal outcome of 12,021 singleton and 3108 twin births after non-IVF-assisted reproduction: A cohort study. *Hum Reprod* 21:1025–1032.
8. Pinborg A., Lidegaard O., Freiesleben N., and Andersen A.N. 2007. Vanishing twins: A predictor of small-for-gestational age in IVF singletons. *Hum Reprod* 22:2707–2714.
9. Hoy J., Venn A., Halliday J., Kovacs G., and Waalwyk K. 1999. Perinatal and obstetric outcomes of donor insemination using cryopreserved semen in Victoria, Australia. *Hum Reprod* 14:1760–1764.
10. Lansac J., Thepot F., Mayaux M.J. et al. 1997. Pregnancy outcome after artificial insemination or IVF with frozen semen donor: A collaborative study of the French CECOS Federation on 21,597 pregnancies. *Eur J Obstet Gynecol Reprod Biol* 74:223–228.

29

IUI-Associated Infection Risks and Preventative Measures

Carin Huyser

Introduction

The reproductive care for a couple includes the screening for infections to provide responsible and safe healthcare according to standard operative procedures, regulations or directives that may differ from country to country. Resources available could influence the range of fertility screening and concurrent diagnostic and therapeutic healthcare decisions, which include scheduling for intra-uterine insemination (IUI) with the husband/male partner's sperm. Measures should be in place to ensure detection, prevention, and where appropriate treatment of infectious organisms to guard predominantly against cross-contamination. Infections originate mostly through biological specimens from patients that harbor infectious conditions, but can also occur through contact with health workers, contaminated laboratory environment, equipment, and storage vessels, as well as materials and supplies utilized during procedures (Figure 29.1). By identifying the potential sources, protective measures can be taken to prevent transmission of pathogens. Multiple targets must therefore be managed to prevent and control contamination of infectious agents in a laboratory setting.[1] One of the primary objectives of any assisted reproduction technology (ART) unit (including the laboratory section responsible for semen processing) should be to recognize, reduce, or possibly eliminate risks for introducing and transmitting pathogens from all internal and external sources.

Three sections will be discussed, as is depicted in Figure 29.1, that is, (i) patient evaluation and screening for microbes, (ii) sperm preparations to reduce infectious agents, and (iii) risk-reduction through the prevention of environmental and procedural contamination in an IUI program. Statements (including published Level of Evidence) and recommendations (Grade Strength) are presented in Tables 29.1 and 29.2, respectively. It should be noted that no Level 1 or 2 evidence is available on the subject, whereby authority or expert-based evidences were referenced.

Discussion

Screening of Patients for Microbes: Detection and Prevention

Work-up of couples prior to ART treatment and handling of human bodily fluids during procedures is generic for all patients, irrespective of the type of ART procedure. Various viral agents such as cytomegalovirus (CMV), hepatitis B, C, D (HBV, HCV, HDV), herpes simplex virus type 2 (HSV-2), human T-lymphotrophic virus (HTLV), and human immunodeficiency virus (HIV) can be transmitted through semen and vaginal secretions.[1] Finances available clearly influence the choice and scope of sexual transmitted infections (STIs) screening, selection of ART procedures, and choice of a private or public ART sector in low to middle-income countries. The practice of routine microbial semen cultures in asymptomatic couples is debatable; however, patients should be routinely screened for HIV, HBV/ HCV as well as other predominantly prevalent STIs, and the laboratory staff notified of the test results,

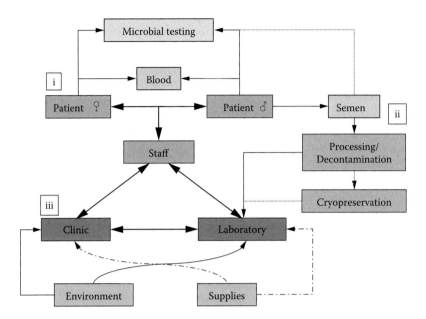

FIGURE 29.1 Elements that influence the prevention of infections during an IUI program: (i) Patient evaluation and screening, (ii) semen sample and sperm processing, and (iii) environmental and procedural factors.

before processing or cryopreservation of any biological specimen.[2] Molecular validation techniques are time consuming and expensive, especially for patients with minimal resources, and limited or no health insurance. Economics and the degree of access to pathology laboratories could hinder regular screening of patients for microbes. ART units should therefore consider the use of rapid tests in comparison to molecular assays for a first-line viral and STI validation, that is affordable with a short time span to perform the tests, interpret, and provide results. The development of point-of-care tests could play a significant role in future infectious disease screening and reproductive health management in resource-constrained countries.[3] Although staff should handle all (blood and) semen samples with extreme care as a biohazard, which could possibly harbor infectious micro-organisms,[4] rapid tests can possibly fast-forward pathology results and ensure that semen samples are always handled in an informed manner.

Microbes are present in approximately 50% of all semen samples obtained by masturbation for diagnostic or therapeutic procedures, with gram-negative species present in only a fraction of samples. Four possible combined or separate approaches when dealing with bacterial contaminants in semen are: (i) strict guidelines are provided (directives on sample collection) to male patients to eliminate skin-contaminants, (ii) appropriate treatment is subsequently prescribed based on susceptible testing of semen, prior to an assisted reproduction procedure (i.e., in comparison to prophylactic antibiotic treatment), (iii) semen washing/processing solutions contain antibiotics, and (iv) the use of a physical mechanism (such as a mechanical device, for example, the ProInsert™, Nidacon, Sweden) combined with density gradient centrifugation (DGC) to reduce microbe recontamination in the processed sperm sample.[3] The sterile collection of semen for microbiological analyses (and therapeutic use) should always be followed, which is urination, washing of hands and genitals with soap followed by thorough rinsing and drying, and ejaculation into a clean labeled specimen container.[4] A nonspermicidal nontoxic polyurethane condom (e.g., Male-FactorPak®, Apex Medical Technologies, California) can be issued to HIV-negative males where semen can only be collected through sexual intercourse,[3] which is preferable to coitus-interruptus where the first sperm-rich portion of a sample may be lost and the semen sample can be contaminated with vaginal flora and cells.[4] Female patients presenting with vulvo-vaginitis caused by *Trichomonas vaginalis*, candidiasis due to *Candida albicans*, and vaginosis as a result of anaerobic bacteria, as well as *Mycoplasma hominis*, *Gardnerella vaginalis* infections, or general urethritis and cervicitis syndromes, should be treated with antibiotics[1] prior to the scheduled IUI cycle. The male partner of the female should be similarly evaluated, screened, and treated prior to an IUI attempt. Also, unnecessary prescription (costs and use) of antibiotics to male patients can be prevented, if comprehensive verbal (and written) instructions on laboratory procedures and guidelines on semen collection are provided prior to the initial semen evaluation, well before the scheduled IUI treatment cycle.[3]

Sperm Preparations to Reduce Infectious Agents

Semen analyses should be performed according to the World Health Organization (WHO) manual for the processing of human semen,[4] taking into account the European Society of Human Reproduction and Embryology guidelines for the preparation of sperm samples for insemination purposes.[2] Tissue grade sterile disposables should be used aseptically in the laboratory, together with density gradients and/or media that has not expired,[2] and has been stored according to the manufacturer's specification for sperm processing.

Sperm preparation techniques using centrifugation to purify sperm from seminal plasma include a simple washing procedure, the direct swim-up technique, and discontinuous density gradient centrifugation. The simple washing procedure usually presents with the highest sperm yield and can be used for semen samples of good quality. The WHO laboratory manual[4] commented that leukocytospermia may indicate the presence of an infection and can be associated with poor sperm quality. Discontinuous gradients, on the other hand, can be standardized and provide superior separation of highly motile spermatozoa from debris, leukocytes, and other cell types. Sperm preparation techniques, however, cannot guarantee a total effectivity to eliminate infectious agents from semen[4] and the risks associated with sperm washing should be discussed with patients.[5] A *Cochrane*-based review by Eke and Oragwu[5] indicated that reports on the use of sperm washing for HIV-seropositive patients, at this time, are only observational in nature. Since no seroconversions were reported in the literature after sperm-washing procedures, it is neither ethical nor legal not to offer the risk-reduction sperm-washing procedures to patients that tested positive for HIV, either in the case of a randomized control study[5] or ART treatment procedure. This overwhelming safety record is supported by evidence obtained from European centers using IUI, *in vitro* fertilization (IVF), and intra-cytoplasmic sperm injection (ICSI) procedures; and published data from ART centers in the United States where ICSI is predominantly preferred as the ART method of choice for HIV-positive males. HIV-regulations, variations in ART treatment modalities, as well as costs of sperm washing and ART procedures (with particular reference to resource-limited countries in Africa) may well contribute to the lack of equivalent randomized trials in this area of ART.[5]

Sperm washing refers to the process whereby spermatozoa are separated from the seminal plasma, in view of the presence of the HIV in the seminal fluid as well as nonsperm cells, and nonattachment to spermatozoa.[5] Even though similar activities such as centrifugation, washing with separation solutions, and the addition of a swim-up technique are incorporated during the processing of semen samples from HIV-seropositive males, the overall sperm-washing technique may vary significantly in different laboratories. The term *sperm decontamination* was introduced[3] to distinguish sperm washing from the decontamination procedure used for samples possibly containing infectious microbes, for example, bacteria, HIV, HCV, and CMV. This entails using a ProInsert™ to facilitate accurate layering of density gradients and the semen sample (Figure 29.2), and to retrieve the purified motile sperm pellet (after centrifugation) via an elongated pipette without recontamination of the sperm pellet with infectious micro-organisms. A final washing step (without an additional swim up) follows where a portion of the purified sperm sample should be tested for HIV-1 proviral DNA and RNA using a sensitive molecular-based technique (e.g., polymerase chain reaction [PCR]).[4] Only HIV-free sperm samples should be made available for IUI. The ProInsert™ provides a biosecure method for the operator, since the contaminated layers (cellular debris, bacteria, and viral-containing fractions) are capped and discarded appropriately as biohazardous waste. It is important to note that over 60% of all neat semen samples from HIV-positive males may test positive for either HIV-1 RNA quantitatively or DNA qualitatively.[3] Validation of results is to ensure that postprocessed sperm samples are not contaminated with, for example, HIV. Results may only be available after 48 hours and this necessitates the need for cryopreservation of the purified sperm[3] using high-security sperm straws and dedicated liquid nitrogen storage tanks.[2]

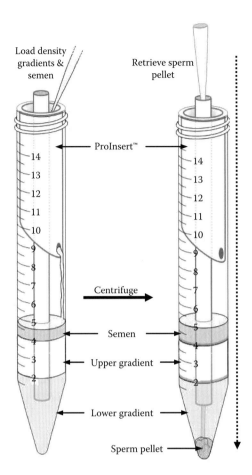

FIGURE 29.2   Schematic presentation of the semen decontamination procedure using a ProInsert™; from layering of gradients and semen to the retrieval of the purified sperm pellet using an elongated micropipette.

Environmental and Procedural Aspects

Contact with contaminants in the working environment, exposure to pathogens in body fluids from patients participating in the ART program or micro-organisms from healthcare staff, will definitely have a negative impact on gamete survival. Exposure of gametes or embryos to pathogenic organisms has the potential to transmit disease to several targets such as the couple under ART treatment, other couples, health workers, a resulting embryo and/or other co-incubating gametes or embryos.[1] Guidelines for good laboratory practices should therefore be followed to promote quality and safety within the ART unit.[2] Policies and procedural documentation will direct patient evaluation, screening, and treatment options in a defined environment according to a standard operative procedure in an IUI program.

Sufficiently qualified and experienced staff should ensure (i) the laboratory facilities are appropriately designed with adequate equipment and disposables to minimize various risks, (ii) establishment of procedures and policies on the safety of staff, (iii) prevention of sample cross-contamination, (iv) enforcing of protective measures when handling body fluids, and (v) mandatory identification and documentation of patients and all biological specimens obtained from patients.[2] The laboratory staff should be rigorously trained in the safe handling of all body fluids. Personnel, with written consent, should also be vaccinated against HBV with a baseline serum result available,[1] and also for other viral diseases for which vaccines are available.[2] Skin breaks should be sealed with waterproof dressings and nontoxic powder-free gloves should be worn at all times, with appropriate barrier precaution in place (clothing, masks, gowns, and goggles).[1,2]

Biosafety for ART procedures are classified as being Level 2, with additional precautions when handling HIV and HBV/HCV-positive samples. It is prudent to ensure separate facilities as well as equipment for semen handling and cryopreservation,[1] however, specimens from patients who tested positive for blood-borne viruses should be processed in dedicated areas with appropriate safety measures.[2] An alternative is the batching or scheduling of seropositive patients to allow sufficient decontamination of the laboratory[2] after semen processing and inseminations. All procedures and manipulation of the semen samples should be performed in Class II biological safety cabinets (BSCs) with vertical laminar flow, using aseptic techniques, and sterile disposables.[1,2] Validation by certification of the BSC should be performed upon installation and thereafter annually, to ensure a microbe-free environment for semen handling (specimen), operators, and the environment.[1] Semen samples should always be centrifuged in sealed buckets or rotors to restrict aerosol formation. Herewith all sharp objects should be handled with extreme care[2] and rather be avoided when handling specimens from patients with blood-borne pathogens. Eating, drinking, and smoking are evidently prohibited in the laboratory, together with restrictive access to authorized staff only.[2] Unhygienic working conditions and waste disposal definitely increases the risk that infections may be transmitted to personnel, patients, cultures, samples, and equipment.

TABLE 29.1

Statements of Chapter 29

Statement	Level of Evidence (LOE)
Patient Screening and Practices	
Infections originate mostly through biological specimens from patients that harbor infectious conditions, but can also occur through contact with health workers, contaminated laboratory environment, equipment, and storage vessels, as well as materials and supplies utilized during procedures	4
All biological specimens (blood and semen samples) must be handled with extreme care as a biohazard, since they are most likely to harbor infectious micro-organisms	4
A nonspermicidal condom should be used rather than the practice of coitus-interruptus, since the latter can result in the loss of the first sperm-rich portion and can contaminate the semen sample with vaginal flora and cells	3
Unnecessary prescription (costs and use) of antibiotics to male patients can be prevented, if comprehensive verbal and written instructions on laboratory procedures and guidelines on semen collection are provided prior to the initial semen evaluation, well before the scheduled IUI treatment cycle	3
Sperm Preparations	
DGC can be standardized and provide superior separation of highly motile spermatozoa from debris, leukocytes, and other cell types	4
Sperm samples contaminated with pathogenic organisms will negatively impact on IUI outcome	4
Sperm-washing techniques are used to prevent partner-to-partner transmission during an IUI procedure	2b
Sperm preparation techniques do not guarantee that HIV is 100% removed from the postprocessed sperm sample of HIV-positive males	2b
A ProInsert™ combined with DGC provide a biosecure method to purify spermatozoa from HIV-positive males	3
No seroconversions of female partners were reported in the literature, at this time, after inseminations with washed sperm from HIV-positive men	2b
Other	
Uncluttered work surfaces, hygienic working conditions, and waste disposal management will reduce the probability of laboratory contamination	4
Protective measures to adhere to while performing ART procedures are designed to protect laboratory personnel and certify aseptic conditions for gametes, zygotes, and embryos	4
Guidelines for good laboratory practices should be followed by trained personnel to promote quality and safety in the ART unit	4

TABLE 29.2

Recommendations of Chapter 29

Recommendation	Grade Strength
Patient Screening	
Patients should be routinely screened for HIV, HBV/HCV as well as prevalent STIs in an IUI program, and laboratory staff should be notified of the test results, before processing or cryopreservation of any semen samples	D
Both male and female patients should be screened for pathogens and treated prior to an IUI attempt	C
ART units should consider the use of rapid tests in comparison to molecular assays for a first-line viral and STI validation	C
Sperm Preparations	
The sterile collection of semen for microbiological analyses and therapeutic use should always be followed	D/GPP
The risk-reduction sperm preparation procedures should be offered to patients that tested positive for blood-borne viruses (HIV/HCV/CMV) as part of an ART treatment procedure	B
A portion of the postprocessed purified sperm sample from HIV-positive males should be tested by RT-PCR for HIV-1 proviral DNA and RNA analyses, and only HIV-free samples should be used for IUI	C
High-security straws and dedicated liquid nitrogen storage tanks should be used to cryopreserve sperm samples after washing/decontamination	D
Healthcare Personnel	
Personnel should be vaccinated against HBV or viral diseases where vaccine is available	D
Ensure all staff are qualified and appropriately trained to handle infectious specimens	D
Protective measures should be enforced when handling body fluids (masks, gowns, and goggles)	D
Skin breaks on exposed skin of staff should be sealed with waterproof dressings and nontoxic powder-free gloves should be worn all the time	D/GPP
Environment/Procedures	
Laboratory facilities should be appropriately designed with adequate equipment and disposables to minimize various risks	D
Semen samples from patients who tested positive for blood-borne viruses should be processed in dedicated laboratory areas with appropriate safety measures	D
All procedures and manipulation of the semen samples for IUI should be performed in Class II biological safety cabinets with vertical laminar flow, using aseptic techniques and sterile disposables	D
All sharp objects should be handled with extreme care and rather be avoided when handling (semen and blood) samples from patients with blood-borne pathogens	D
Access to the laboratory should always be restricted to protect the workplace integrity and to prohibit eating, drinking, as well as smoking within the laboratory	D/GPP

The laboratory should be clear of unnecessary clutter and all work surfaces and floors must be cleaned (decontaminated) daily.[1]

An assisted reproduction laboratory is a complex structure geared toward the promotion of optimal cell survival and culture, not only for gametes and embryos, but also for viruses and bacteria.[1] Introduction of infectious conditions into the IUI program can be prevented if the origin of the contaminant can be identified, contained, or removed. ART practices can thus avert disasters by knowing the infectious demography of patients visiting the unit, and to follow guidelines for good clinical and laboratory practices to improve quality and safety within the unit.

REFERENCES

1. Elder K., Baker D.J., and Ribes J.A. 2005. Part II: Infections in reproductive medicine and Part III: Infections and the assisted reproductive laboratory. In: *Infections, Infertility and Assisted Reproduction*. United Kingdom: Cambridge University Press.
2. Magli M.C., Van den Abbeel E., Lundi K., Royere D. et al. 2008. Revised guidelines for good practice in IVF laboratories. *Hum Reprod* 23:1253–1262.

3. Huyser C. and Fourie J. 2010. Sperm only please: Prevention of infections in an assisted reproduction laboratory in a developing country. *F, V & V in ObGyn* Monograph:97–106.

4. World Health Organisation. 2010. *WHO Laboratory Manual for the Examination and Processing of Human Semen*, 5th ed. Geneva: WHO Press.

5. Eke A.C. and Oragwu C. 2011. Sperm washing to prevent HIV transmission from HIV-infected men but allowing conception in sero-discordant couples. *Cochrane Database Syst Rev* 1:CD008498.

30

Cancer and Semen Preservation

Roelof Menkveld

Introduction

In early reports on semen banking, the cryopreservation of semen for cancer patients for use in artificial insemination was thought to be pointless if motility was <40% and sperm concentration was <20 million spermatozoa per ml, due to unacceptable low chances for conception. Even if the semen quality before freezing was better than the above-mentioned criteria, pregnancy rates were still very poor. Therefore, as a result, even today many oncologists consider semen cryopreservation for cancer patients as insufficient and not worthwhile to perform.[1]

With improved techniques semen cryopreservation has now become an important part of the routine work of most andrology or assisted reproductive laboratories. There are two main reasons for cryopreservation of semen; one is for the use in donor semen-related procedures and the second for the purpose of fertility preservation in males, also known as autoconservation.[1] In this chapter the emphasis will be on storage of semen for autoconservation in male cancer patients only, with reference to the effects of cryopreservation on semen parameters and sperm functions and the use of cryopreserved semen in practice. There is still a perception by the public at large and professionals in the field that semen autoconservation is a routine and simple process. Yet semen storage requires a number of unique skills from a multi-disciplinary team of oncologists, nurses, counsellors, scientists, and embryologists in order to provide a quality service to the patient.[2]

Cancer and Male Infertility

Men presenting with infertility have an increased risk of testicular cancer. It has been reported that testicular cancer dominates as the leading cancer in men between 15–34 years of age. Many men presenting with infertility are in the age group of 30–35 years, the same as men with the highest prevalence of testicular cancer, and therefore are high-risk cancer patients. Testicular cancer is very common in American men with a prevalence of 4.84/100,000 men and 1/100,000 in black men. The risk increases to 9.92/100,000 for men in the age group 30–34. Over the last 30 years, there has been a significant increase in the frequency of testicular cancers (especially seminomas) and a decrease of semen quality. One of the reasons may be the increase of in utero environmental exposure to endocrine disruptors modulating the genetically determined fate of the primitive gonads resulting in the testicular dysgenesis syndrome, which may result in decreased semen parameters and cancer. Better understanding of common mechanisms involved in infertility and testicular cancer, and the scientifically driven evidence-based treatment options should improve the quality of life in young men faced with this potentially life-threatening disease.[3]

Conservation of Fertility in Male Cancer Patients

For patients to undergo cancer therapy with alkylating agents or radiotherapy, the semen must be collected before the patient commences with any therapy in order to decrease the risk of mutagenesis during spermatogenesis and genetic alternations of spermatozoa.

Semen Quality in Cancer Patients

Different reports are published regarding semen parameters of males with cancer. In most instances similar semen qualities are reported in men with and without cancer while some reports indicate that semen quality may be compromised.[1]

Effect of Cancer Treatment on Semen Parameters and Male Fertility

It is well known that the kind of cancer and the kind of treatment, that is, chemotherapy with cytotoxic agents or radiotherapy, may have different effects on spermatogenesis and eventually on the fertility status of the male. The effect may be permanent or temporary, but it is seldom found that the male will recover to his full fertility potential. Studies indicate that one year post-radiotherapy treatment, 16% of men who were initially diagnosed with normozoospermia presented with oligozoospermia and 20% were still azoospermia. However, spermatogenesis in patients who received cancer treatment can improve over the next 5 years.[1]

Availability of Semen Cryopreservation for Male Cancer Patients

A few surveys have been published in the literature reporting on the availability of semen cryopreservation services and the actual usage once the semen samples have been stored. A survey performed in Australia and New Zealand among pediatric oncology centers reported that from the 13 questionnaires sent out to different centers, 12 centers responded. All 12 centers offered semen cryopreservation but only 9 of the 12 centers offered counseling as a routine procedure. Likewise, in a survey among oncologists in the United States, 91% of the responders agreed that semen conservation procedures should be offered but only 27% offered the service sometimes while 10% always offered the service.[1] A problem area may be the variation in various practices and the background of unresolved medical, legal, and ethical issues. For this reason development of specific guidelines and rules is essential.[2]

Counseling and Ethical Issues—Informed Consent

When using both therapeutic and experimental techniques informed consent is essential. In presenting the various therapies, the men have the right to know their options concerning fertility preservation as well as the risks and costs involved. Therefore, the ideal situation should be that counseling for a candidate for fertility preservation should be rendered by a multiple expert team (as mentioned), all guided by written protocols that can be shared with patients.[4]

Effects of Cryopreservation on Semen Parameters and Sperm Functions

It is well known that cryopreservation of semen does have a negative effect on semen parameters and sperm function, especially on sperm motility. On average only 50% of the motile spermatozoa will survive freezing and thawing with a corresponding reduction in vitality while damage of sperm structure and function also occurs. Alternations in acrosome structure as well as shrinkage of sperm nuclei and cytoplasmic membranes with loss of plasma membrane integrity and the concurrent reduction of intact acrosomes and consequently a reduction in (pro)acrosin activity has been observed. Due to the addition of the cryoprotectant there is also a reduction in the sperm concentration. The effect of cryopreservation on semen parameters of cancer patients is in the same order.[1]

Use of Cryopreserved Semen in Practice

Only a small percentage of males who cryopreserved their semen samples will eventually use the stored semen samples. The usage of cryopreserved semen varies between 30% to less than 10% of the stored samples but in many centers it may be as low as 5% or less.[1]

Time of Storage

Semen stored under appropriate conditions will show no deterioration of sperm quality with time and has successfully been used after 20 years of storage.[1]

Pregnancy Rates with Stored Semen

Best pregnancy rates with artificial insemination performed with cryopreserved donor semen are no different from those achieved with fresh semen and pregnancy rates range from 15 to 25% per month, or cycle of treatment. However, pregnancy rates of 7–12% per month are more common. Rates are often related to post-thaw sperm quality, timing of insemination, and are particularly influenced by recipient factors such as age of the women and tubal or uterine disorders. Evidence suggests that there is no increase in abnormal pregnancy outcomes after the use of cryopreserved semen for intra-uterine insemination (IUI). The rates for spontaneous abortion of 13%, major birth defects of about 1%, and the sex ratio of 51:49, males:females, are similar to those of spontaneous pregnancies.[1]

Long-Term Follow-Up of Use of Cryopreserved Semen Samples

Magelssen et al.[5] reported their experience over a 20-year time span with semen cryopreservation in testicular cancer patients. If offered, 50% of men with testicular cancer were interested in semen cryopreservation. For the period 1983 to 2002, 30.4% (422/1,388) of new patients diagnosed with testicular cancer asked for semen cryopreservation. All these patients were followed-up for post-treatment paternity. A total of 29 (7%) used their cryopreserved semen at least one time for assisted reproductive technology (ART), of which 55.1% (16/29) achieved pregnancies. They also reported that 17% (67/393) of the men with cryopreserved semen fathered at least one child without the use of their frozen semen while 21% (205/966) of patients without cryopreserved semen fathered a child.

Emotional Aspects of Semen Cryopreservation

Although a considerable number of testicular cancer patients who had cryopreservation of their semen samples achieve fatherhood without the use of their frozen semen samples, the knowledge that these samples were available had a positive psychological impact.[5]

A questionnaire completed by 66 cancer patients with cryopreservation of their semen revealed that only 50% banked sperm on their own initiative and 60% were worried about their fertility status. After chemotherapy, 70% wanted a child but none of the patients wanted to use their cryoperserved semen for insemination if found that spermatogenesis was restored, as reflected by a positive semen analysis. As much as 80% of the patients reported that sperm banking helped them in the battle against cancer, especially those who asked for cryopreservation on their own initiative. Most patients recommended cryopreservation to other patients. Sperm cryopreservation before cancer chemotherapy, therefore, helps in the emotional battle against cancer.[6]

TABLE 30.1

Statements of Chapter 30

Statement	Level of Evidence (LOE)
Sperm cryopreservation before cancer chemotherapy helps in the emotional battle against cancer	1a
Cryopreserved semen samples can still be used after more than 20 years of storage	1a
Semen cryopreservation is still not offered as a standard service in most centers treating male cancer patients	1b
Best IUI results with cryopreserved semen can be similar to IUI results with fresh semen	2a
Semen cryopreservation should be performed before the start of cancer treatment	1a
Cancer treatment has a permanent or temporary negative effect on semen parameters and males will seldom recover their full fertility potential after treatment	1a

TABLE 30.2

Recommendations of Chapter 30

Recommendation	Grade Strength
Semen cryopreservation should be offered to all male cancer patients	A
Semen cryopreservation should be performed before the start of cancer treatment	A
Before semen cryopreservation, the patient should be counseled by a multi-task team	B
More research on semen cryopreservation is needed, especially for young adolescents and boys	B

Future Developments in Preservation of Male Fertility

Semen cryopreservation can only help those cancer patients with some degree of complete spermatogenesis. However, there are a great number of patients and young adolescents and boys where spermatozoa are not available. For boys, testicular stem cell banking is the only way forward.[7] The existence of spermatogonial stem cells in the testis offers clinically relevant options for preservation and restoration of male fertility with the possibilities of male germ cell transplantation and testicular tissue grafting.[1]

Conclusions

Semen cryopreservation is an essential procedure for male cancer patients. Although the request rate is low, if used, pregnancy rates are compatible with other IUI procedures. The storage of semen from cancer patients should be offered, after sufficient consultations, to all cancer patients before cancer treatment because of the positive mental role it can play (see also Tables 30.1 and 30.2). If not offered, legal action can be taken against the treating institution.

REFERENCES

1. Menkveld R. 2010. Bank your future: Insemination and semen cryopreservation. *F V and V ObGyn* Monograph:68–73.
2. Pacey A.A. and Eiser C. 2011. Banking sperm is only the first of many decisions for men: What healthcare professionals and men need to know. *Hum Fertil* 14:208–12.
3. Paduch DA. 2006. Testicular cancer and male infertility. *Curr Opin Urol* 16:419–28.
4. Patrizio P. and Caplan A.L. 2010. Ethical issues surrounding fertility preservation in cancer patients. *Clin Obstet Gynec* 53:717–26.
5. Magelssen H., Haugen T.B., von Düring V., Melve K.K., Sandstad B., and Fosså S.D. 2005. Twenty years experience with semen cryopreservation in testicular cancer patients: Who needs it? *Europ Urol* 48:779–85.

6. Saito K., Suzuki K., Iwasaki A., Yumura Y., and Kubota Y. 2005. Sperm cryopreservation before cancer chemotherapy helps in the emotional battle against cancer. *Cancer* 104:512–4.
7. Tournaye H., Goossens E., Verheyen G., Frederickx V., De Block G., Devroey P., and Van Steirteghem A. 2004. Preserving the reproductive potential of men and boys with cancer: Current concepts and future prospects. *Hum Reprod Update* 10:525–32.

31

Preconception Gender Selection: Laboratory Aspects

Lars Björndahl

Introduction

A general problem affecting studies on variation in natural and induced gender outcome is that with few exceptions, reports are based on small, selected populations. A ratio different from 0.50 could be due to random variation, or from bias in the selection of cases. For a correct interpretation of available data it is essential to take into consideration that factors which influence the natural sex selection are far from completely understood. The live birth sex ratio in humans does not appear to be a simple reflection of the X-Y ratio in semen. Other factors, for example, uterine environment, may also contribute to the final sex ratio. Thus, validation of sex selection methods cannot be based exclusively on data from "enriched" sperm populations, but must include the evaluation of pregnancies resulting from the treatment with such sperm populations.

Methods

In this review of published studies, preconception methods possibly useful for patients undergoing intra-uterine insemination (IUI) or *in vitro* fertilization (IVF) will be discussed. It is in this limited clinical area that studies have been performed and published.

Sperm Selection

Laboratory methods for sex selection before insemination have primarily been developed for domestic animals. The validation of these methods is less demanding in the large-scale insemination programs in the cattle breeding industry. Separation of Y- or X-bearing spermatozoa has been the goal for methods developed also for humans. The selection methods for preconception use generally consist of a passage of sperm through different gradients or of flow cytometry. Also methods based on immunological techniques and electrophoresis have been investigated, but without showing signs of clinical value.

The theoretical basis for the procedures to separate spermatozoa with different sex chromosomes is the expected differences in sperm characteristics (size, dry mass, and DNA content). There are, however, other factors complicating the situation for human spermatozoa. For instance, the huge variability in sperm head size within each semen sample is much larger than the small differences that are due to the X- and Y-chromosomes. Therefore, the two populations overlap to a considerable extent and make the separation far from complete.

Gradient Methods

Different methods to select highly motile spermatozoa devoid of seminal plasma have been developed to increase success in various forms of assisted reproductive techniques (ART). Some have been claimed to change the sex ratio at birth. The more common variants have been centrifugation through gradient layers of albumin, varying density preparations as Percoll™ and Ficoll™, or microbead suspensions like Sephadex™. In addition, methods based on sperm migration through media of different composition (swim up) have been described.

	Desired Gender[a]	Method[b]	Initial Group[c]	No. of Treated Couples[d]	Leaving Study without Conception	Couples Remaining	Not Conceiving	Number of Conceptions	Preterm Ending, Gender Unknown[e]	Preterm, Male Gender[f]	Preterm, Female Gender[g]	Molar Pregnancy	Normal Pregnancies	MALES[h]	FEMALES[h]	Still Pregnant[i]	Not Counted or Unknown
Dmowski et al. 1979[6]	Y	A	37	37		37	27	10		1				6	2	2	
Beernink and Ericsson 1982[7]	Y	A		66	22	44	14	30	3				15	12	4	5	
	Y	AC											5	1	5		
	Y	A											46	38	9		
	Y	AC											7	1	7		
	Y	A												19	7		
Corson et al. 1983[8]	X	S	3					1					2		1	1	
Corson et al. 1984[9]	Y	A		79				40	3	1	1		30	28	7	1	
	Y	A											26	19	7		
	X	S		19				12	1				11	2	8	1	
Jaffe et al. 1991[10]	Y	A	162	112									23	13	10		
	X	AC	87	50									14	3	11		
	CY		107	107									23	14	9		
	CX												17	11	6		
Beernink et al. 1993[11]	Y	A												749	285		
	X	AX												60	133		
Check and Katsoff 1993[12]	Y	M												25	5		
	Y	P												19	17		
	C													13	13		
Rose and Wong 1998[13]	Y	A	184	112				31	6					15	4		3
Khatamee et al. 1999[14]	X	M											15	2	13		
	Y	M											37	33	4		

[a] X = Female, Y = Male; C = Control group
[b] A = Albumin gradient; AX = Albumin gradient for X-sort; AC = Albumin gradient + Clomid treatment; S = Sephadex gradient; M = modified swim-up; P = Percoll filtration; C = Control
[c] Number of patients coming for initial consultation for gender selection
[d] Number of patients that were treated
[e] Abortions, ectopic pregnancy
[f] Spontaneous abortions
[g] Miscarriage
[h] Including preterm ended pregnancies with known gender
[i] According to statement in publication

FIGURE 31.1 Summary of published, peer-reviewed reports (found in searches at Medline) on clinical outcome (pregnancies) after albumin or other gradient separation methods.

Albumin Gradients

A fairly simple method with an albumin gradient was published by Ericsson et al.[1] The exact mechanism for a possible selection of spermatozoa in an albumin gradient is not known and the validity of the method has been challenged. It may be that the quinacrine dye could cause false positive, stained cells due to the high concentrations of albumin. Still, there are several reports on the sex of conceptions and children born after insemination with spermatozoa selected by albumin gradients (Figure 31.1). However, several studies by independent clinics have not been able to verify that the albumin gradient method actually changes the ratio between X- and Y-bearing spermatozoa although a few have given some support.[2–4] The main objection concerning the validity of the positive studies is the lack of results from independent clinics, not performing sex selection on a commercial basis. Furthermore, patients who have withdrawn from studies arc usually not included. Conversely, there are no clinical studies that have disproved that the gender outcome may be altered by the albumin gradient separation method. However, from the point of prevention of inheritance of severe diseases, the efficiency can be questioned: there is a 15–30% possibility to achieve the *undesired* gender—a risk that is not acceptable when the problem is a severe sex-linked genetic disease.

Other Gradients

Commercially available gradients like Percoll, Ficoll, or Sephadex for sperm selection do not appear to give clinically significant results in controlled studies.[4] Only a low number of couples with clinical pregnancy have been retrospectively reported to give clinically important results for density gradient centrifugation combined with sperm migration in a medium (Figure 31.1). In contrast, other studies have not revealed important differences in the ratio between X- and Y-spermatozoa when validating the methods with molecular genetic techniques.

Flow Cytometry

Flow cytometry for the selection of X- and Y-bearing spermatozoa is based on the difference in DNA staining by the dye Hoechst 33342. Selected spermatozoa are then used for ART. The validation of the efficiency of the sperm selection has predominantly been done with polymerase chain reaction (PCR) or FISH on selected spermatozoa, or by biopsy of the developing embryo (pre-implantation genetic diagnosis, PGD). The difference in the DNA content of X- and Y-bearing spermatozoa in humans is the smallest among animals. Still, purities of X- and Y-bearing sperm of 70–90% have been reported.

The main safety issue with the sorting technique is the potential hazards inflicted on the sperm DNA. Hoechst 33342 binds to DNA and emits energy (light) when hit by a laser beam that in itself conveys energy to the DNA. The excess energy can cause damages to the DNA. However, the probability of one major, easily discernible defect to occur repeatedly in different individuals is almost zero. In contrast, an increase of different damages would only be possible to differentiate from the *background noise* after the birth of several thousand individuals after performing the technique.

Spermatozoa from humans are exposed to lower concentrations of Hoechst 33342 and for a shorter time compared to domestic animals. It must, however, be taken into account that the lower exposure used for human sperm reflects a relatively easily accessible sperm chromatin. This means that the exposure of the human sperm DNA to potentially damaging compounds can be even greater than that used for domestic animals.

Results and Discussion

According to a published report, linked to the license owner of the flow cytometry system Microsort®, a study on human sperm sorting has been ongoing between 1994 and 2007 comprising 3,952 couples and 5,871 sperm sort events. Sorting sperm to enrich X-bearing spermatozoa (X-sort) gave 87.9% purity of X-bearing spermatozoa. Sorting sperm to enrich Y-bearing spermatozoa (Y-sort) gave 73.4% purity of Y-bearing spermatozoa (as validated with FISH) on the level of spermatozoa. The result expressed as gender of born children the X-sort resulted in 92.0% girls and for Y-sort 81.5% boys. The data on child gender included an unknown number of IVF/ICSI cycles where PGD was used in addition to the sperm sorting. Thus, the total result is a mix of IUI cycles with only sperm sort, and IVF/ICSI cycles where some cycles have included PGD, and the data therefore do not reveal a pure sperm sort effect. For IUI there were 3,629 sorts performed (unknown number of couples). The pregnancy rate for IUI cycles was about half that of the IVF/ICSI cycles (15.6% cf. 32.0%). No PGD could be offered to IUI patients, and separate data were not provided. For all treatment cycles a total of 801 births were achieved from 1,125 clinical pregnancies. Out of these 801 births, 760 medical records were reviewed: 2.6% had major malformations, 6.1% minor congenital, and 3.0% showed variants. The author concluded that the frequency of major malformations did not differ significantly from that of the general population.

Conclusions

The efficiency of gradient procedures has not been scientifically validated by independent clinics. Although the flow cytometry sorting method appears to be a reliable method for preconceptual sex selection, there are some issues that must be considered. The equipment, the expertise, and the technology involved in flow cytometry are expensive. The MicroSort technology is only available under a commercial license. All sorts are performed on the premises of GIVF in the United States. However, pregnancy rates are good, thus allowing the use of sperm in IUI. This widens the availability of the technology and does reduce costs. However, although rather successful with regard to sorting, the risk for *error* can be 10–30% unless PGD is used in connection with IVF/ICSI. This must be regarded as unacceptable for a couple aiming to avoid a severe sex-linked disease, and it makes the method less suitable when IUI is considered (see also Tables 31.1 and 31.2).

The full extent of the risk for inducing inheritable damages to the sperm DNA by the flow cytometry sorting procedures is not completely covered by present scientific investigations. There are well-grounded theoretical implications that irradiation energy and radicals generated may cause damages in the DNA. The available numbers of individuals and generations born, and the level of evaluation of

TABLE 31.1

Statements of Chapter 31

Statement	Level of Evidence (LOE)
Sperm selection for IUI with gradients may result in increased probability for a certain gender, but the probability for the other gender is still significant	3
Sperm sorting using DNA binding compound Hoechst 33342 can increase the probability for the birth of a child with a specific gender after IUI but the probability for the other gender is still significant, especially when PGD is not possible to use	2b
The potential risks for DNA damage using DNA binding compound Hoechst 33342 have not been fully investigated	4

TABLE 31.2

Recommendations of Chapter 31

Recommendation	Grade Strength
Sperm selection using gradients is not a suitable choice before IUI to avoid inheritance of serious genetic diseases	C
Sperm selection by flow cytometry sorting before IUI is not recommended as a means to avoid inheritance of a serious genetic disorder	B
Sperm selection by flow cytometry sorting before IUI is at present not recommended as a means for social gender choice (*family balancing*) since the risk for the individual without congenital factors is unknown but potentially severe	GPP

possible increases in DNA damage in these individuals, cannot rule out that other, less obvious damages have occurred.

Future research must consider both the actual outcome of gender in children born after sperm selection *and* the potential risks for damage to future generations when, for example, chemical compounds, combined with a high supply of energy (e.g., laser), are used to target the sperm and its DNA content in relation to the risk one wishes to avoid (e.g., a severe genetic disease or family "unbalance").

REFERENCES

1. Ericsson, R.J., C.N. Langevin, and M. Nishino 1973. Isolation of fractions rich in human Y sperm. *Nature* 246(5433):421–4.
2. Flaherty, S.P. et al. 1997. Albumin gradients do not enrich Y-bearing human spermatozoa. *Hum Reprod* 12(5):938–42.
3. De Jonge, C.J. et al. 1997. Failure of multi-tube sperm swim-up for sex preselection. *Fertil Sterl* 67(6):1109–14.
4. Vidal, F. et al. 1993. Sephadex filtration and human serum albumin gradients do not select spermatozoa by sex chromosome: A fluorescent *in-situ* hybridization study. *Hum Reprod* 8(10):1740–3.
5. Karabinus, D.S. 2009. Flow cytometric sorting of human sperm: MicroSort clinical trial update. *Theriogenology* 71(1):74–9.
6. Dmowski, W.P. et al. 1979. Use of albumin gradients for X and Y sperm separation and clinical experience with male sex preselection. *Fertil Steril* 31:52–57.
7. Beernink, F.J. and R. Ericsson. 1982. Male sex preselection. *Fertil Steril* 38:493–495.
8. Corson, S.L., F.R. Batzer, and S. Schlaff. 1983. Preconceptual female gender selection. *Fertil Steril* 40:384–385.
9. Corson, S.L. et al. 1984. Sex selection by sperm separation and insemination. *Fertil Steril* 42:756–760.
10. Jaffe, S. et al. 1991. A controlled study for gender selection. *Fertil Steril* 56:254–258.
11. Beernink, F.J., W.P. Dmowski, and R.J. Ericsson. 1993. Sex preselection through albumin separation of sperm. *Fertil Steril* 59:382–386.
12. Check, J.H. and D. Katsoff. 1993. A prospective study to evaluate the efficacy of modified swim-up preparation for male sex selection. *Hum Reprod* 8:211–214.
13. Rose G.A. and A. Wong. 1998. Experiences in Hong Kong with the theory and practice of the albumin column method of sperm separation for sex selection. *Hum Reprod* 13: 146–149. Erratum (Rose and Wong 1998): *Hum Reprod* 13:1414.
14. Khatamee M.A. et al. 1999. A controlled study for gender selection using swim-up separation. *Gynecol Obstet Invest* 48:7–13.

32

Preconception Sex Selection: Ethical Evaluation

Guido Pennings

Introduction

Several methods of preconception sex selection have been presented over the years, going from diets, over timing of intercourse, to sperm separation. This chapter will only consider the method with scientifically proven efficacy, that is, sperm separation through flow cytometry.

Ethical Arguments

The normative ethical theories can be separated into two large types: deontological and consequentialist theories. These theories answer the question: What should we do? In other words: which act is good or right?

Deontological Considerations

The deontological theories focus on the relationship between the act, decision, and so forth, and the relevant moral rule, principle, and so on. An act is right when it is in agreement with the rule. There are many arguments against sex selection from a deontological position. The first one is that wanting to determine the sex of one's child demonstrates the wrong attitude of the parents toward their future child. Parents who want to choose characteristics of their child (the *designer baby* argument) do not respect the child as an autonomous person. By choosing the sex, parents violate the rule that "good parents accept their child as it comes." The second counterargument is that sex selection is morally wrong because it is sexist, that is, the choice shows that the parents value one sex as inherently better than the other. Third, from a broader philosophical perspective, sex selection is condemned because it is *unnatural*. This perspective is part of a more negative, or cautious, attitude toward technology and medicalization. Nature regulates things in such a way that about as many boys as girls are born and human intervention may disturb this balance. A final argument is that a child is a gift from God and should be accepted as such. However, not all deontological arguments oppose sex selection. The most important deontological argument in favor of sex selection is the principle of respect for reproductive autonomy: people have the right to decide whether or not to have children, the timing, the health (through genetic testing), the number, and the gender composition of their family. Generally speaking, deontological arguments seem to dominate the public debate. The main problem with deontological arguments is that they are based on an ideological basis (religion, worldview, etc.) that is not shared by everyone.

A crucial distinction for the ethical evaluation is that between medical and nonmedical applications. Medical applications, that is, when there is a high risk of transmitting a sex-linked genetic disease, are considered ethically acceptable by the overwhelming majority. Social or psychological reasons, like parental preference or societal appreciation of one sex, are not accepted. However, the distinction between medical and nonmedical applications is not as clear-cut as generally presented. First, the more genetic information we have about a person, the more people will be able to advance a medical reason for selecting the sex of their child. Whole genome screening will provide huge amounts of information and almost every person will have a genetic condition with either a different penetrance in one sex (e.g., bilateral renal agenesis) and/or a different expression in the sexes (e.g., ankylosing spondylitis). How skewed should the sex ratio be before we call it a medical reason? How different should the expression in the sexes be before it is a medical application? Second, there are intermediate reasons, for example, to avoid that one's children have to face difficult reproductive decisions in the future, that may also justify sexing.[1]

Preconception sex selection would be inappropriate in case of a high risk for a serious genetic disease. The reliability of the technique (92% for daughters and 82% for boys) is insufficient. Certainty about the future child's sex would be required and, at the moment, only preimplantation and prenatal genetic diagnosis can fulfill this condition. Still, a two-step process may be the least burdensome for the woman. In the first step, sperm selection could be used to increase the percentage of low risk (usually female) embryos. In the second step, preimplantation or prenatal testing is performed but, because of the first step, there is an increased chance of having good quality embryos of the right sex to replace and a lower chance of having to recur to an abortion after prenatal testing. So preconception sex selection may have its role in a broader procedure for medical reasons.

An interesting shift in the evaluation of the technique is raised by the comparison with alternative techniques, that is, postconception and/or postimplantation techniques. Most people prefer preconception techniques because it avoids the contentious issue of the status of the embryo and the problem of abortion. At present, many couples in countries with a clear sex preference recur to prenatal testing followed by abortion. One can assume that many of these couples, and especially the women, would prefer preconception methods. The question then becomes whether it would not be morally preferable to offer preconception techniques in such countries, further restricted to a family-balancing framework.[2] The same question may arise very soon in developed countries after the introduction of noninvasive prenatal testing. This technique will enable parents to determine the sex of the fetus at a very early stage in the pregnancy. Couples who want to choose the sex of their child will be able to do so without explanation or justification because the intervention is covered by the abortion laws. This raises the question of whether we should stick to the principle of not allowing sexing regardless of the method or whether we should adopt a more flexible position taking into account the desires of some parents and the harm involved in postconception interventions.

Utilitarian Considerations

The second group of theories can be brought together under the header of consequentialism. Utilitarianism is the most popular among these theories. A utilitarian believes that an act, decision, and so forth, is good when it generates more utility (expressed as happiness, quality of life, or well-being) than any other act that person could have performed. Applied to our problem, sex selection is good if it generates more happiness for all people involved than not selecting the sex of one's child. Empirical data are indispensable for this decision. The findings from the human sciences (psychology, sociology, etc.,) allow a more objective basis for the evaluation but it is still very complicated. First, there is paucity of data regarding the consequences of sexing. Numerous statements are made on these points by both opponents and proponents without any evidence whatsoever. Opponents state that a child will feel psychologically harmed when it will find out that its sex has been chosen by its parents or that children who are born with the wrong sex after treatment will suffer more. Proponents suggest that children born with the desired sex will be happier and that the family will be more harmonious. Second, this approach demands the inclusion of all stakeholders (parents and society at large) and not just the child. Given the dynamics within a family and given the complex interactions between society and technology, a comprehensive global balance will be hard to construct.

When looking at the consequences, two distinctions should be made: (1) between micro-level consequences for the individuals and their family, and macro-level consequences for society, and (2) between medical and psychosocial consequences. An important difficulty for the consequentialist position at the moment is a so-called catch-22: the defenders of preconception sexing have to prove that the technique is safe for the resulting children but they cannot prove this because they are not allowed to apply the technique without proof.

Medical and Psychosocial Consequences

Although specific concerns exist regarding the safety of sperm separation through flow cytometry, the technique has been used for years in animals without adverse findings. Limited data in humans are available and these data are reassuring for short-term safety: there is no increased malformation rate in the children.[3] The issue of safety and efficacy related to the introduction of new techniques in medicine is highly complicated. The general conditions are animal studies, preclinical embryo studies, clinical trials in humans, and follow-up studies. These steps are ethically relevant since they assure, as far as possible, the well-being of patients and offspring.

In addition to medical information, psychological and social follow-up is also needed. Such information is now obtained for other controversial changes such as new family forms (lesbian couples) and modifications of specific rules (donor anonymity). If we ever want to have an idea about the consequences of preconception sex selection for children, parents, and society at large, we need to allow a limited number of cases and do the follow-up. There is more, however. When a technology is available, we also need to study the families in which parents have a strong wish for a specific sex and no sexing is allowed. The legal prohibition of an existing technique makes the lawmaker responsible for the consequences of its nonapplication. Although the evidence is very limited, there is one study that indicates that there are negative consequences for children who did not have the sex desired by the parents.[4]

Micro-Level and Macro-Level Consequences

In addition to the direct familial consequences of sex selection, we should also take into account the larger effects on society. This not only refers to the possibility of a skewed sex ratio.[5] Sociological evidence from countries with large-scale applications of sex selection in favor of boys shows disastrous effects on many aspects of society, including general development and family building. Two additional ethical and ideological aspects should be scrutinized: the impact of sex selection on (a) sex role stereotyping, and (b) the status of women. These broad societal concerns should be taken seriously and should be part of follow-up research. It would be unacceptable if we find out years from now that for instance sexing technology reinforced rigid gender roles while most societies simultaneously adopted other measures to discourage this evolution (see also Tables 32.1 and 32.2).

TABLE 32.1

Statements of Chapter 32

Statement	Level of Evidence (LOE)
There is widespread approval of preconception sex selection for medical reasons	4
Most international committees and many countries condemn sex selection for nonmedical reasons	4
Family balancing is frequently presented as a compromise between reproductive autonomy of the would-be parents and societal concerns	4

TABLE 32.2

Recommendations of Chapter 32

Recommendation	Grade Strength
The appropriate steps for introducing new techniques into the field of medically assisted reproduction should be started for preconception sex selection	D
Follow-up studies should be set up to determine the social and psychological consequences for the child and its parents of (a) allowing sex selection and (b) prohibiting sex selection	D
Studies should be organized to determine the social consequences for society at large, including the impact on ethical convictions such as the equality of the sexes	D
Public campaigns and educational programs should be established in gender-biased societies to address the social norms and structural issues underlying sex discrimination	D

REFERENCES

1. De Wert G. and Dondorp W. 2010. Preconception sex selection for non-medical and intermediate reasons: Ethical reflections. *Facts, Views and Vision in Obstetrics and Gynecology* 2:267–277.
2. Pennings G. 1996. Ethics of sex selection for family balancing—Family balancing as a morally acceptable application of sex selection. *Human Reproduction* 11:2339–2343.
3. Karabinus D.S. 2009. Flow cytometric sorting of human sperm: Microsort clinical trial update. *Theriogenology* 71:74–79.
4. Stattin H. and Klackenberg-Larsson I. 1991. The short- and long-term implications for parent-child relations of parents' prenatal preferences for their child's gender. *Developmental Psychology* 27:141–147.
5. Dahl E., Beutel M., Brosig B., Grussner S. et al. 2006. Social sex selection and the balance of the sexes: Empirical evidence from Germany, the UK, and the US. *Journal of Assisted Reproduction and Genetics* 23:311–318.

33

Factors Affecting the Success of IUI: Implications for Developing Countries

Hasan N. Sallam

Introduction

The term *developing countries* is a technical term used by the World Bank to define countries according to their Gross National Income (GNI) per capita. The list includes 152 countries with a low or middle GNI per capita. An alternative definition is that used by the UNDP (United Nations Development Programme) for the *least developed countries*, which includes 50 countries, of which 33 are in Africa and nine in Asia.

Infertility in developing countries possesses specific aspects, which may not apply to the developed world due to etiological, financial, and cultural differences. The financial and psychological burdens of infertility are also more pronounced and are confounded by many cultural and logistical obstacles to fund infertility services and train the personnel, and access to these services may be difficult even if they exist.

Consequently, intra-uterine insemination (IUI) offers many advantages as a treatment option for patients in developing countries over other forms of assisted reproduction. It is easy to learn, requires less equipment, and is less expensive and less invasive. It is associated with reduced psychological burden and the couple compliance is usually good. In addition, the risk of ovarian hyperstimulation syndrome (OHSS) is reduced and the rate of multiple pregnancies is also lower when performed with natural cycles, clomiphene citrate, or low-dose gonadotrophin stimulation protocols.

Optimizing IUI for Developing Countries—Overview of the Evidence

Optimizing an IUI program for a developing country requires the simplification and cost reduction of the following steps:

- The stimulation protocol
- The timing of insemination
- The method of semen evaluation
- The sperm preparation techniques
- The insemination technique
- The number of inseminations per cycle
- Dealing with infected semen samples (particularly HIV and/or hepatitis B or C)

The success rate of IUI is a function of the number of follicles developing in response to stimulation. In a meta-analysis by Van Rumstke et al., the absolute pregnancy rate was 8.4% for mono-follicular and 15% for multi-follicular growth and this difference is statistically significant in the presence of two, three, and four follicles (LOE 1a).[1]

Consequently, most infertility specialists perform IUI in stimulated cycles and clomiphene citrate (CC) stimulation is particularly suited for developing countries. Ombelet et al. found that patients treated with CC and IUI achieved an overall cycle fecundity (CF) and take-home baby rates (THB) of 14.6% and 9.9%, respectively. The cumulative CF and THB (per couple) after three cycles were 30.6 and 21.1%, respectively. These findings were similar in all patients except when the insemination motile count was $< 1 \times 10^6$ and the strict morphology score was <4% normal forms (LOE 2b).[2]

Similarly, there is no evidence that conventional CC-HMG protocols increase the pregnancy rate over simpler regimens. Dhaliwal et al. compared the conventional CC + HMG daily (from day 8) protocol to a minimal stimulation protocol of CC + one HMG injection (150 IU on day 9) in patients undergoing IUI and found no significant difference in clinical pregnancy rate per cycle. More importantly, the cost of the treatment cycle was U.S. $63.50 for the minimal stimulation cycle versus U.S. $216.50 in the conventional stimulation cycle (LOE 2a).[3]

Various methods for timing IUI have been proposed, but none of them seems to be superior to the others. In a *Cochrane Review* by Cantineau et al., no significant differences in live birth rates were found between different methods of timing IUI: hCG versus LH surge, urinary hCG versus recombinant hCG, and hCG versus GnRH agonist. In addition, all the secondary outcomes analyzed showed no significant differences between treatment groups. The authors concluded that the choice of timing should be based on hospital facilities, convenience for the patient, medical staff, costs, and dropout levels (LOE 1a).[4]

There is no evidence that computer-assisted semen analysis (CASA) is more accurate than conventional semen analysis. Hofmann et al. found that trained andrologists are as good as CASA in evaluating sperm morphology (LOE 2a).[5] Training courses for laboratory technicians on semen evaluation are conducted regularly with help of WHO in various parts of the world in order to standardize the procedure and many of these courses are conducted in developing countries, particularly in Africa.

Evidence reveals that no sperm preparation technique is superior to any other. A *Cochrane Review* conducted by Boomsma et al. including 262 couples found no significant difference in clinical pregnancy rates or the miscarriage rate between swim-up and a gradient or wash and centrifugation technique in the five RCTs (LOE 1a). There was no evidence of a difference in the miscarriage rate in two studies comparing swim up versus a gradient (LOE 1a).[6]

Different catheters have been used for IUI with various claims of success. It has been suggested that soft catheters may be less traumatic to the uterine cervix or to the endometrium. However, in a recent *Cochrane Review*, Van der Poel et al. found no significant difference regarding the choice of catheter type in live birth rates, clinical pregnancy rates, or the rate of miscarriages (LOE 1a).[7]

There is also no advantage of performing IUI twice over once in the same cycle. In the *Cochrane Review* of Cantineau et al., no significant difference was found between the single and double IUI groups in the probability for clinical pregnancy (LOE 1a).[4]

Finally, regarding HIV which is endemic in many developing countries in Africa and Asia, it has now been established that methods of preparing the sperm in which the seminal plasma is removed by washing and sperm are separated from the other cellular elements of the sperm (e.g., centrifugation on discontinuous gradients) can reduce the viral load up to an undetectable level. In a recent meta-analysis including 3,900 IUI cycles in HIV serodiscordant couples (with a seronegative female partner), the pregnancy rates per cycle were 18%, the cumulative pregnancy was 50%, and the abortion rate was 15.6%. No seroconversions in women or newborns were detectable at birth or after 3 to 6 months (LOE 2a).[8]

Discussion

It is clear from the above-mentioned evidence that various steps involved in IUI can be simplified for use in developing countries without compromising the efficiency of the technique. These steps include the use of mild stimulation protocols in the form of clomiphene citrate with or without the addition of one ampoule of gonadotrophins and timing the insemination with ultrasound folliculometry and hCG injection. The simplest sperm preparation technique can be used, that is, the swim-up method when the sperm count is adequate and the wash/centrifugation method when the count is low. Gradient techniques should be reserved for infected samples. Inexpensive rigid catheters perform as well as more expensive ones and one insemination per cycle is as good as two. Finally, proper dealing with HIV infected samples can totally prevent seroconversion.

Conclusions

IUI is a simple, affordable, and effective treatment for infertility in indicated cases and is particularly suited to developing countries. Randomized trials have shown that IUI can be successfully performed in patients with limited resources using simple approaches. Evidence has shown that many of the steps involved can be simplified without compromising its efficiency (see also Tables 33.1 and 33.2).

TABLE 33.1

Statements of Chapter 33

Statement	Level of Evidence (LOE)
The absolute pregnancy rate is higher with multi-follicular compared to mono-follicular growth	1a
CC + IUI is an efficient method of infertility treatment unless the insemination motile count is $<1 \times 10^6$ with a strict morphology score of <4%	2b
CC + IUI is associated with a low risk of multiple pregnancies and no moderate or severe OHSS	2b
There is no significant difference in clinical pregnancy rates between minimal stimulation protocols of CC + one HMG and conventional CC-HMG protocols used with IUI, while the first method is cheaper	2a
There is no significant difference in live birth rate between different methods of timing IUI	1a
There is no significant difference between conventional evaluation of sperm morphology and computer-assisted methods	2a
There is no significant difference in clinical pregnancy rates between different methods of sperm preparation	1a
There is no significant difference in live birth rates, clinical pregnancy rates, or the rate of miscarriages between soft and rigid insemination catheters	1a
There is no significant difference in clinical pregnancy rates between single and double inseminations in the same cycle	1a
In HIV infected semen samples, sperm washing and centrifugation on discontinuous gradients reduces the viral load to an undetectable level	2a

TABLE 33.2

Recommendations of Chapter 33

Recommendation	Grade Strength
CC + IUI is an effective and affordable method for the treatment of infertility and is particularly suited to developing countries	B
Folliculometry + HCG should be used for IUI timing	B
Conventional semen analysis by trained personnel are as good as CASA for semen sample evaluation	B
In low resource settings, the simplest and affordable sperm preparation technique should be used as it is as good as other methods	A
The simplest affordable catheter can be used for IUI as it is associated with similar pregnancy rates to more expensive catheters	A
A single properly timed insemination per cycle is sufficient and is as good as double insemination	A
In HIV discordant couples, semen samples should be treated with centrifugation on discontinuous gradients without fear of seroconversion	B

REFERENCES

1. Van Rumste M.M., Custers I.M., Van der Veen F. et al. 2008. The influence of the number of follicles on pregnancy rates in intrauterine insemination with ovarian stimulation: A meta-analysis. *Hum Reprod Update* 14:563–657.
2. Ombelet W., Vandeput H., Vande Putte G. et al. 1997. Intrauterine insemination after ovarian stimulation with clomiphene citrate: Predictive potential of inseminating motile count and sperm morphology. *Hum Reprod* 12:1458–1463.
3. Dhaliwal L.K., Sialy R.K., Gopalan S. et al. 2002. Minimal stimulation protocol for use with intrauterine insemination in the treatment of infertility. *J Obstet Gynaecol Res* 28:295–299.
4. Cantineau A.E., Janssen M.J., and Cohlen B.J. 2010. Synchronised approach for intrauterine insemination in subfertile couples. *Cochrane Database Syst Rev* April 14 (4):CD006942.
5. Hofmann G.E., Santilli B.A., Kindig S. et al. 1996. Intraobserver, interobserver variation of sperm critical morphology: Comparison of examiner and computer-assisted analysis. *Fertil Steril* 65:1021–1025.
6. Boomsma C.M., Heineman M.J., Cohlen B.J. et al. 2007. Semen preparation techniques for intrauterine insemination. *Cochrane Database Syst Rev* October 17 (4):CD004507.
7. Van der Poel N., Farquhar C., Abou-Setta A.M. et al. 2010. Soft versus firm catheters for intrauterine insemination. *Cochrane Database Syst Rev* November 10 (11):CD006225.
8. Vitorino R.L., Grinsztejn B.G., de Andrade C.A. et al. 2011. Systematic review of the effectiveness and safety of assisted reproduction techniques in couples serodiscordant for human immunodeficiency virus where the man is positive. *Fertil Steril* 95:1684–1690.

34

SWOT Analysis of Accessible IUI in Developing Countries, Resource-Poor Settings, and Primary Care Centers

Willem Ombelet and Sheryl Vanderpoel

Introduction

As mentioned in Chapter 3, we have to realize that intra-uterine insemination (IUI) should only be offered to a couple if the success rate after IUI clearly exceeds the probability of a treatment independent pregnancy in that couple. Therefore, a good prognosis in clinical decision making should be made based on adequate and reliable prediction models.

If assisted reproduction is needed, it is generally accepted that IUI can be offered as a first-line treatment in nontubal factor cases of unexplained infertility and moderate male factor subfertility before using the more invasive and expensive IVF/ICSI techniques of assisted reproduction. Scientific validation of this strategy is difficult because the literature is rather confusing and not conclusive. If IUI is promoted as a first-line treatment, it is necessary to evaluate cost–benefit analyses, complication rates, and invasiveness of techniques as well as couple compliance, especially within resource-poor settings.

IUI has been proven to be easier to perform, less invasive, and less expensive than other more complex methods of assisted reproduction.[1] Effectiveness of IUI compared to IVF in case of unexplained and moderate male infertility has been documented.[2] Risks are minimal provided the multiple gestation incidence can be reduced to an acceptable level and efforts are made to decrease horizontal transmission of sexually transmitted infections (STIs), including HIV.

Therefore, increasing interest in IUI is undoubtedly associated with the refinement of techniques for the preparation of washed motile spermatozoa.[3,4] Semen-washing procedures can remove prostaglandins, infectious agents, antigenic proteins, nonmotile spermatozoa, leukocytes, and immature germ cells. This may enhance sperm quality by decreasing the formation of free oxygen radicals after sperm preparation. The final result is an improved fertilizing capacity of the sperm *in vitro* and *in vivo*.

In developing countries and within low resource settings, reflection on the implementation and use of IUI as a first-line treatment for most cases of nontubal infertility should be considered. Costs are minimal, training can be easily accomplished, quality control possible, and severe complications are minimal by using optimal semen-washing procedures and by avoiding gonadotrophins for ovarian stimulation as much as possible in order to prevent multiple gestations and the occurrence of ovarian hyperstimulation syndrome (OHSS).

The major complication of assisted reproductive technology remains the high incidence of multiple pregnancies, responsible for a significantly increased maternal and child mortality and morbidity. This will automatically burden the treatment because of the high costs of caring for premature newborns and infants as a result of the "induced" multiple gestations. Therefore, careful monitoring is essential and cancellation of the insemination procedure, escape-IVF, and follicular aspiration before IUI are reasonable options if multiple gestations could result due to identification of multiple follicular development.

Natural cycle IUI, clomiphene citrate, and minimal dose (step-up) regimen with gonadotrophins are valuable options in order to prevent maternal and child adverse events.

Ovarian hyperstimulation syndrome may complicate all methods of treatment within which gonadotrophins are used. OHSS appears to be a rare serious adverse event after OH/IUI compared to IVF due to the fact that lower-dose stimulation protocols are more often used within IUI programs.[1]

Globally, healthcare cost consciousness has become an integral component of policy and is also important for health decision makers. Evidence related to the cost and effectiveness of infertility treatment exists, but most studies deal with procedures associated with IVF. Published data comparing cost of IVF versus IUI indicate that initiating treatment with IUI appears to be more cost-effective than IVF in case of unexplained, nontubal factors, and moderate male subfertility, although this interpretation is not consistent across all studies.[2,5,6,7]

SWOT Analysis

Strength

IUI is a simple and noninvasive technique, which can be performed without expensive infrastructure with a reasonable cumulative live birth rate within three or four cycles, making this method of assisted reproduction very appealing for developing countries and low resource settings, as well as for programs providing universal health coverage.

The costs for training health providers as well as the direct and indirect costs are minimal compared to IVF/ICSI. The use of affordable and safe washing techniques coupled with the value of natural cycle or clomiphene citrate stimulation also adds to the value of IUI since assisted reproductive technologies such as IVF/ICSI are either unavailable or very costly, and within low resource settings only within reach of the happy few who can afford it. For almost all religions and societies, artificial insemination with husband's semen is permissible, another advantage for introducing IUI as a first-line treatment option.

Weaknesses

IUI programs do require a minimal infrastructure with dedicated well-trained personnel. For example, a basic infertility service should be capable of offering the following services: basic infertility work-up including HSG (hysterosalpingography), semen analysis, follicular scanning, postcoital testing (PCT) in addition to ovulation induction with or without IUI. In some developing countries, even these minimal requirements cannot be fulfilled.

The low live birth rate per treatment cycle (between 5 and 10%) is another disadvantage for IUI, especially for couples who live within rural areas and have to travel far to get the IUI treatment.

It is well known that in many resource-poor countries, especially in sub-Saharan Africa, most subfertile couples suffer from tubal factor infertility and/or severe male factor infertility. In both cases, doing IUI is not indicated, IVF or ICSI are the only treatment options.[8]

Opportunities

Transmission of life threatening STIs such as HIV, HCV, and hepatitis B constitute particular risks in developing countries. It is estimated that nearly 40 million people worldwide are infected with HIV. Most HIV patients are residents of developing countries, of reproductive age, and many maintain a desire to have children. Many studies have shown that appropriate sperm processing coupled with IUI or vaginal insemination may reduce the risk of HIV transmission. Semen-washing techniques appear to be safe and effective, offering HIV-serodiscordant couples and couples where both partners are infected an opportunity to have children within an environment where services are available to provide antiretroviral therapy and HIV-monitoring.[4]

According to a *Cochrane Review* on semen preparation techniques for IUI, there is insufficient evidence to recommend any specific or a best-practice preparation technique,[3] however, the specific conditions in developing countries or countries with high burdens of STI/HIV were not taken into account in the interpretation. In developing countries and low resource settings, the simplest high-quality semen preparation technique should be used. In areas with a low prevalence of STI/HIV the swim-up method can be used when the sperm count is adequate (>5 million/ml), while a wash and centrifugation method should be used when the count is low (<5 million/ml). Gradient techniques should be used in all countries and within all settings with a high prevalence of STI/HIVs and a high rate of seminal infections.

The use of a novel innovative semen-washing procedure which combines multiple density gradients and trypsin for removing STIs including HIV and hepatitis C virus and viral particles from semen seems very promising.[4]

A basic infertility service can be affordably established for the implementation of IUI programs within developing countries, lower resource and primary care settings worldwide. Infertility service clinics within primary care settings should be equipped with low-cost and easily serviceable devices and commodities taking into consideration the local problems (e.g., fluctuating voltage, frequent power cuts, unavailability of servicing facilities, irregular supply of consumables, etc.).

Providing basic infertility care requires a simple ultrasound machine with a vaginal probe (with an electric battery), a simple binocular microscope, an inexpensive temperature box, a basic centrifuge, a laboratory pipette set, and a refrigerator, in addition to two UPS (uninterrupted power supply) units.[9]

Threats

To address issues of maternal and child mortality and morbidity, and limitations for many facilities worldwide to handle multiple births, premature neonates and OHSS (which can be fatal) infertility care must follow best-practice guidelines.

In this regard, as guidelines in infertility are just being developed by WHO, the best practice for IUI procedures should attempt to prevent multiple pregnancies. This means that the use of natural cycle (NC) IUI, especially in cases of cervical factor and moderate male subfertility, is recommended. CC ovarian stimulation can safely be applied in case of unexplained infertility with the benefit of being very cheap when compared to ovarian stimulation with gonadotrophins. However, the cumulative ongoing pregnancy rate when using NC-IUI or CC-IUI is significantly lower compared to IUI after ovarian stimulation with less affordable recombinant Follicle Stimulating Hormone (rec-FSH) or (purified) urinary gonadotrophins.

Nevertheless, the strategy of using NC-IUI or CC-IUI as a first-line treatment in most cases of nonobstructive subfertility is of outstanding importance for developing countries, low resource settings, and primary care settings worldwide. Furthermore, best practice would dictate that ultrasound monitoring of IUI cycles is practiced if ovarian stimulation is used. This would allow for a decrease in serious adverse events by implementing a cycle cancellation or a follicle aspiration if three or more follicles with a mean diameter of >13 mm are present.

Semen collection can be difficult, especially for persons adhering to religious recommendations where masturbation is to be avoided if possible, and this means that in these areas coitus interruptus and the use of a specific condom is the preferred method for semen collection. IUI with donor semen (AID) can also be restricted under various situations within some settings.

Conclusions

IUI is a simple, noninvasive, and affordable treatment modality, which can be used as a first-line treatment in nontubal factor subfertility cases which include mild and moderate male subfertility. The technical requirements necessary and the current scientific evidence on the success and complication rates provide sufficient evidence to promote IUI as a first-line treatment modality in developing countries, low resource setting, and primary care centers worldwide. Classical algorithms for the diagnosis and treatment of male and female infertility (WHO guidelines in development) should be followed and preference should be given to those treatment modalities with the lowest complication rates, best obstetrical and child outcomes, affordable costs, and cultural acceptance (see Tables 34.1 and 34.2).

In this view, a proper diagnosis is needed to select the couples in which IUI can be promoted as the best first-line treatment. It can be concluded that in a large group of subfertile couples it may be unwise to initiate treatment with the expensive IVF and/or ICSI methods without trying out IUI (see also Table 34.1).

TABLE 34.1

Statements of Chapter 34

Statement	Level of Evidence (LOE)
IUI could be offered as a first-line treatment in case of nontubal factor, unexplained, and moderate male factor subfertility, provided the multiple gestation incidence can be reduced to an acceptable level and provided at least one fallopian tube is patent	1b
Multiple gestations are the most important complication associated with IUI after gonadotrophin stimulation and should be avoided as much as possible	2a
Semen decontamination through sperm processing can prevent transmission of life threatening STIs and other infectious agents, which constitute a high risk in developing countries and lower resource settings	2a

TABLE 34.2

Recommendations of Chapter 34

Recommendation	Grade Strength
IUI could be provided as a first-line therapy to all patients providing at least one patent tube and an inseminating motile count (IMC) after sperm preparation of more than 1.0 million	B
When ovarian stimulation is used, a careful monitoring of the IUI cycle is needed to avoid multiple pregnancies	C
Gradient techniques should be used in all settings with a high prevalence of STI/HIVs and/or a high rate of seminal infections	B

TABLE 34.3

SWOT Analysis of Artificial Insemination in Developing and Resource Poor Countries

Strength	IUI is a simple and noninvasive technique
	IUI techniques and methods are easy to learn, thus training is minimal
	Direct and indirect costs are arguably minimal compared to IVF/ICSI
	A reasonable cumulative live birth rate after three or four IUI cycles
	Severe adverse events and complications are rarely seen
	IUI with partner's semen is permissible within most societies
Weaknesses	In some developing countries even minimal requirements of infrastructure and trained personnel is not prioritized and thus cannot be fulfilled.
	The low live-birth rate per cycle of IUI compared to IVF
	IUI cannot be used in case of tubal factor infertility or severe male infertility, which was identified (1985) as a significant burden of infertility in many developing countries
Opportunities	Transmission of STIs, including HIV, can be prevented through techniques employed together with IUI
	The setting up of a primary care level infertility service center, which could easily be adapted to include IUI techniques, is not expensive and within reach of many developing countries and within lower resource settings
Threats	Avoiding complications such as multiple pregnancies and OHSS is crucial
	An inability to implement IUI techniques, if masturbation and IUI with donor sperm are restricted or denied.

REFERENCES

1. Ombelet W., Puttemans P., and Brosens I. 1995. Intrauterine insemination: A first-step procedure in the algorithm of male subfertility treatment. *Hum Reprod* 10 (Suppl.1):90–102.
2. Goverde A.J., McDonnell J., Vermeiden J.P. et al. 2000. Intrauterine insemination or *in vitro* fertilisation in idiopathic subfertility and male subfertility: A randomised trial and cost-effectiveness analysis. *Lancet* 355:13–18.
3. Boomsma C.M., Heineman M.J., Cohlen B.J. et al. 2007. Semen preparation techniques for intrauterine insemination. *Cochrane Database Syst Rev* 17:CD004507.
4. Loskutoff N.M., Huyser C., Singh R. et al. 2005. Use of a novel washing method combining multiple density gradients and trypsin for removing human immunodeficiency virus-1 and hepatitis C virus from semen. *Fertil Steril* 84:1001–1010.
5. Pashayan N., Lyratzopoulos G., Mathur R. 2006. Cost-effectiveness of primary offer of IVF versus primary offer of IUI followed by IVF (for IUI failures) in couples with unexplained or mild male factor subfertility. *BMC Health Serv Res* 6:80.
6. ESHRE Capri Workshop Group. 2009. Intrauterine insemination. *Hum Reprod Update* 15:265–277.
7. Wordsworth S., Buchanan J., Mollison J. et al. 2011. Clomifene citrate and intrauterine insemination as first-line treatments for unexplained infertility: Are they cost-effective? *Hum Reprod* 26:369–375.
8. Cates W., Farley T.M., and Rowe P.J. 1985. Worldwide patterns of infertility: Is Africa different? *Lancet* 14; 2(8455):596–598.
9. Sallam H.N. 2008. Infertility in developing countries—Funding the project. *Hum Reprod* (Suppl 1): 97–101.

35

Summary: Levels of Evidence of All Statements

Levels of Evidence Used in Statements

1a	Systematic review and meta-analysis of randomized controlled trials
1b	At least one randomized controlled trial
2a	At least one well-designed controlled study without randomization
2b	At least one other type of well-designed quasi-experimental study
3	Well-designed non-experimental descriptive studies, such as comparative studies, correlation studies, or case studies
4	Expert committee reports or opinions and/or clinical experience of respected authorities

TABLE 2.1

Statements of Chapter 2

Statement	Level of Evidence (LOE)
If antisperm antibodies are present, semen preparation for IUI with an additional medium to elude the antibodies leads to a better fertilization capacity of spermatozoa	2a
The postcoital test should not be part of the fertility work-up	1b
The medical history can differentiate between women at low or at high risk for bilateral tubal pathology	2b
Identification of those women at highest risk for bilateral tubal pathology is best obtained by combining the patient characteristics with CAT and HSG results	2a
Routinely testing for tubal pathology is not cost-effective	2b

TABLE 3.1

Statements of Chapter 3

Statement	Level of Evidence (LOE)
In couples with a relatively good prognosis ($>30\%$) of a treatment independent pregnancy, IUI should be postponed for at least 6 months	1b

TABLE 4.1

Statements of Chapter 4

Statement	Level of Evidence (LOE)
In couples with a cervical factor subfertility, IUI in natural cycles significantly increases the probability of conception	1b
In couples with a relatively good prognosis for spontaneous pregnancy, IUI should not be applied too soon	1b
The total number of motile sperm inseminated has the ability to predict failure: in other words, when less than 0.8–5 million motile sperm are inseminated, pregnancies hardly occur	1a
When a male factor is present, there is insufficient evidence to conclude whether IUI is effective or not	1a
IUI in natural cycles has no significant beneficial effect over expectant management when the subfertility of the couple is unexplained	1a
In couples with unexplained subfertility, the combination of ovarian hyperstimulation and IUI significantly improves live birth rates	1a
When the total motile sperm count before sperm preparation has an average value above 10 million, defined as a mild male factor, mild ovarian hyperstimulation might be added	1b
In case of mild endometriosis (AFS grade 1 or 2) couples should be treated as couples with unexplained subfertility and patients might benefit from IUI in combination with mild ovarian hyperstimulation	1b
Mild ovarian hyperstimulation for IUI should result in the release of 2 to 3 oocytes	1a

TABLE 5.1

Statements of Chapter 5

Statement	Level of Evidence (LOE)
In case of immunologic infertility, adding 2% albumine to the buffering medium upon sperm retrieval is useful	4
IUI is the first choice before proceeding to IVF/ICSI in case of immunologic infertility	2a

TABLE 6.1

Statements of Chapter 6

Statement	Level of Evidence (LOE)
Female age is the only relevant predictor of the probability of pregnancy in IUI treatment	1b
A sharp decline of IUI success rate is observed in women over the age of 40 years, presumably related to oocyte quality	1b
The benefit of OH in IUI treatment remains unclear in older women	1b

TABLE 7.1

Statements of Chapter 7

Statement	Level of Evidence (LOE)
Increased male age seems to be associated with a decline in semen volume, sperm motility and sperm morphology but *not* with sperm concentration	2a
Semen parameters start to decline after 35 years of age	1b*
Paternal age seems to have no profound effect when the female partner is younger than 35 years	2b
A synergistic adverse effect seems to exist when the female partner is older than 35 years beyond a male age over 35 years	2a
Oxidative stress-induced mtDNA damage and nuclear DNA damage in aging men may put them at a higher risk for transmitting multiple genetic and chromosomal defects	2b

* From Kühnert B. and Nieschlag E., 2004, *Hum Reprod Update* 10(4):327–39; Stewart A.F. and Kim E.D., 2011, *Urology* 78(3):496–9; Tournaye H., 2009, In: *Reproductive Aging,* London: RCOG Press, 89–94; De La Rochebrochard E., McElreavey K., and Thonneau P., 2003, *J Androl* 24(4):459–65.

TABLE 8.1

Statements of Chapter 8

Statement	Level of Evidence (LOE)
Obesity is associated with lower oocyte yield with gonadotrophin stimulation, lower clinical pregnancy rates, and increased pregnancy loss in patients undergoing IVF	2b
In women undergoing gonadotrophin-IUI treatment, fecundity rates are higher in obese patients, even when controlling for women with Polycystic Ovarian Syndrome (PCOS)	3
In women undergoing gonadotrophin-IUI treatment, miscarriage rates are not significantly higher in patients who are obese, compared to women with normal BMIs	3
Decreasing BMI prior to starting a gonadotrophin cycle has not been shown to improve fecundity rates	3

TABLE 9.1

Statements of Chapter 9

Statement	Level of Evidence (LOE)
The success rate of IUI is improved with a morphology score of more than 4% normal forms, a TMCS of more than 5 million and an initial total motility of more than 30%	2a
IUI is an acceptable first-line treatment with an IMC of more than 1 million	2a
If the morphology score is more than 4%, IUI can be performed with an acceptable success rate even if the IMC is less than 1 million	3
The influence of sperm parameters on IUI outcome is influenced by other parameters such as female age and number of follicles obtained after ovarian stimulation	3

TABLE 10.1

Statements of Chapter 10

Statement	Level of Evidence (LOE)
SPTs significantly increased the probability of conception after IUI in couples with male subfertility	1b
ROS can be detrimental for the fertilizing potential of the spermatozoa	2b
IUI outcomes showed to be optimal after 2 days of ejaculatory abstinence	2a
The sample needs to be transported to the laboratory at body temperature	2b
Semen samples need to be produced in sterile containers that have been tested for reprotoxicity	2a
Semen preparation needs to commence as soon as possible after liquefaction of the sample	2b
If the prepared spermatozoa are to be *stored* after the sperm preparation before the IUI, it is advised to use a *sperm buffer* (e.g., HEPES medium)	3
If the IUI is to be performed soon after sperm processing, a bicarbonate buffered-medium can be used throughout the entire process	3
Concerning laboratory outcomes (e.g., semen parameters): the DGC is shown to be superior to the swim-up and wash technique (improvement of morphological normal spermatozoa with grade A motility and normal DNA integrity, reduced concentrations of ROS and leukocytes, less chromatin and nuclear DNA anomalies, better nuclear maturation rates, improved acrosome reaction, and higher hypo-osmotic swelling test reaction)	2a
Concerning clinical outcome (pregnancy rates) after IUI: there is no clear evidence of which SPT is superior	1a
Selection based on sperm surface charge did not lead to any improvement in fertilization rates or embryo quality following ICSI. The Zeta potential method was reported in one study to increase fertilization, implantation, and pregnancy rates, although not significant	2a
Nonapoptotic sperm selection by MACS resulted in spermatozoa with higher motility and less apoptosis, higher embryo cleavage, and higher pregnancy rates. Fertilization or implantation rates were not higher.	2a

TABLE 11.1

Statements of Chapter 11

Statement	Level of Evidence (LOE)
There is no evidence that shorter intervals for the various steps of IUI (collection-preparation; preparation-insemination; and collection-insemination) are associated with a better prognosis	2a
There have been no randomized studies on this topic	1

TABLE 12.1

Statements of Chapter 12

Statement	Level of Evidence (LOE)
The pregnancy rate per cycle is highest in the first three treatment cycles	1b
Couples with mild male subfertility, unexplained fertility problems, or mild endometrioses show acceptable cumulative ongoing pregnancy rates after six cycles of IUI with OH	1b
After the third treatment cycle, ongoing pregnancy rates per cycle remain stable up to the ninth treatment cycle	2a

TABLE 13.1

Statements of Chapter 13

Statement	Level of Evidence (LOE)
Perifollicular blood flow correlates with the maturity of each follicle	2
Perifollicular flow velocity (PSV) above 10 cm/sec or visualization of power Doppler flow more than ¾ around the circumference of the follicle increases the probability of there being a good quality egg following hCG or LH surge	2
Endometrial thickness reflects estrogen levels produced by growing follicle(s)	1
There is no correlation between endometrial thickness and pregnancy rate but an ET less than 6.3 mm is associated with poor receptivity	2
Triple layer endometrial morphology with spiral artery invasion of the endometrium on power Doppler is more predictive of pregnancy than endometrial thickness alone	3

TABLE 14.1

Statements of Chapter 14

Statement	Level of Evidence (LOE)
With regard to pregnancy rates there is no significant difference between timing IUI with hCG injection or urinary LH surge detection	1a
In natural cycles, timing of IUI with LH surge detection in serum revealed a significantly higher pregnancy rate compared to timing with hCG triggering	1b
The optimal time interval between hCG injection and IUI seems to be between 12 and 36 hours	1b
Double IUI does not result in higher pregnancy rates compared with single IUI treatment in women with unexplained subfertility undergoing ovarian hyperstimulation	1a
Double IUI results in higher pregnancy rates compared with single IUI in couples with male factor subfertility	1a
In cycles with multi-follicular development, double IUI does not enhance live birth rates significantly compared with single IUI	1b

TABLE 15.1

Statements of Chapter 15

Statement	Level of Evidence (LOE)
IUI/OH increases ongoing pregnancy rates compared to ICI/OH in TDI	1a
ICI by using a cervical cap increases pregnancy rates compared to standard ICI by straw	1b
Adding OH to inseminations for TDI results in high multiple pregnancy rates	3

TABLE 16.1

Statements of Chapter 16

Statement	Level of Evidence (LOE)
Spermatozoa reach the fallopian tube as soon as 2 minutes after insemination[2–5,7]	2b
10 to 15 minutes immobilization subsequent to IUI, with or without ovarian stimulation, significantly improves cumulative ongoing pregnancy rates and live birth rates[1,6]	1b

TABLE 17.1

Statements of Chapter 17

Statement	Level of Evidence (LOE)
IUI in combination with (mild) ovarian hyperstimulation has been proven effective in couples with unexplained subfertility	1a
IUI in combination with (mild) ovarian hyperstimulation seems effective in couples with minimal to mild endometriosis	1b
IUI in combination with (mild) ovarian hyperstimulation seems effective in couples with mild male subfertility defined as an average total motile sperm count above 10 million	1b
The goal of ovarian hyperstimulation should be the development of two to three dominant follicles	1a
Gonadotrophins used for ovarian hyperstimulation in IUI programs are more effective compared to clomiphene citrate	1a
Doubling the daily dose of gonadotrophins from 75 IU to 150 IU does not result in improvement of treatment outcome while it significantly increases the chances of achieving a multiple pregnancy	1a
Aromatase inhibitors used for ovarian hyperstimulation are, compared with CC, not more effective while being more expensive	1a
Spontaneous LH surges occur frequently in stimulated IUI cycles and might result in lower pregnancy rates	2
Both GNRH agonists and antagonists are not (cost-) effective in ovarian stimulation/IUI programs	1a
The use of luteal support with vaginally applied progesterone in stimulated IUI cycles might increase pregnancy rates but more randomized trials are warranted	1b
The probability of achieving a twin pregnancy in stimulated IUI cycles is approximately 10% while triplets occur in less than 1% of the pregnancies	3

TABLE 18.1

Statements of Chapter 18

Statement	Level of Evidence (LOE)
Luteal phase support using vaginal progesterone improves live birth rates in IUI cycles stimulated with low-dose gonadotrophins in couples with unexplained subfertility	1b
Luteal phase support with vaginal progesterone does not seem to improve pregnancy rates in normo-ovulatory women stimulated with clomiphene citrate for IUI	1b

TABLE 19.1

Statements of Chapter 19

Statement	Level of Evidence (LOE)
For nontubal subfertility, the results indicate no clear benefit for FSP over IUI	1a
After exclusion studies where a Foley catheter was used, FSP resulted in significantly higher pregnancy rate compared to standard IUI	1a

TABLE 20.1

Statements of Chapter 20

Statement	Level of Evidence (LOE)
PAF/IUI improves per cycle and cumulative pregnancy rates in couples with unexplained subfertility	1b

TABLE 21.1

Statements of Chapter 21

Statement	Level of Evidence (LOE)
Lower levels of seminal oxidative stress marker such as 8-hydroxy-2'-deoxyguanosine (8-OHdG) in men whose partners are undergoing IUI cycles is significantly associated with higher pregnancy outcomes	2a
Seminal leukocytospermia is associated with high semen oxidative stress and poor IUI pregnancy outcomes	2a
Factors such as prolonged abstinence time, advanced paternal age which are associated indirectly with high sperm oxidative stress burden are significantly related to poor IUI pregnancy outcomes	3
High sperm DNA damage is associated with low IUI pregnancy rates	2a
Sperm processing methods and use of frozen sperm enhances spermatozoal generation of ROS	2b
The fertilizing potential of frozen sperm is lower than that of freshly ejaculated sperm due to cryopreservation-induced sperm dysfunction and OS	1a
Chronic endometritis is associated with impaired female reproductive performance, possibly due to inflammatory mediators, such as cytokines, eicosanoids, nitric oxide, and OS	4

Note: IUI: intrauterine insemination, ROS: reactive oxygen species, and OS: oxidative stress.

TABLE 22.1

Statements of Chapter 22

Statement	Level of Evidence (LOE)
Primary treatment with IUI compared to immediate IVF is more cost-effective	1a
In couples with unexplained infertility, treatment-independent pregnancies can occur at a reasonably high rate	1b
IUI with clomiphene citrate followed by IVF improves time to pregnancy compared to IUI with clomiphene citrate followed by IUI r-FSH	1b

TABLE 23.1

Statements of Chapter 23

Statement	Level of Evidence (LOE)
The donor should be of legal age and, ideally, less than 40 years of age, because increased male age is associated with a progressive increase in the prevalence of aneuploid sperm	2a
The results to be expected are around 23% pregnancy rates in IUI using mild ovarian hyperstimulation; pregnancy rates in IVF using donor sperm are around 45%	3
Unexpected transmission of genetic diseases using donor sperm is a real possibility	4
All donors should be screened for karyotype, since the frequency of balanced translocations is around 2 per 1,000 tested individuals	2a
Inhalation of N_2 vapors may inadvertently cause a decrease in O_2 concentration, leading to loss of consciousness, cerebral harm, and even death	2a

TABLE 24.1

Statements of Chapter 24

Statement	Level of Evidence (LOE)
Family relationships and psychological development of children are normal	3
Social stigmatizations influence well-being of family members negatively	3
Most children want (identifying) donor information	3

TABLE 25.1

Statements of Chapter 25

Statement	Level of Evidence (LOE)
Discontinuation during conventional fertility treatment or in between conventional treatment and ART is about 9%	3
Most important reasons for discontinuation of conventional fertility treatment are rejection of treatment and relational problems	3
Doctors have difficulties adhering to guidelines for conventional fertility treatment	3

TABLE 26.1

Statements of Chapter 26

Statement	Level of Evidence (LOE)
In stimulated IUI cycles with 3 to 4 follicles the multiple pregnancy rate increased without substantial gain in overall pregnancy rate	1a
Multi-follicular growth, woman's age and estradiol levels are risk factors for HOMP after stimulated IUI cycles	1b
HOMPs are more likely to occur in the first three treatment cycles	1c

TABLE 27.1

Statements of Chapter 27

Statement	Level of Evidence (LOE)
Pregnancy is more likely to occur with two follicles than with one[a]	1a
The risk of multiple pregnancies for two follicles as compared to mono-follicular growth increases by 6%[a]	1a
Higher pregnancy rates are obtained in IUI when combined with gonadotrophins compared to anti-estrogen[b]	1a
Doubling the dose of gonadotrophins does not increase the pregnancy rate[b]	1a

[a] From Van Rumste et al., 2008, *Hum Reprod Update* 6:563–70.
[b] From Cantineau and Cohlen, 2011, *Cochrane Database Syst Rev* 6:CD005356.

TABLE 28.1

Statements of Chapter 28

Statement	Level of Evidence (LOE)
Singleton and twin pregnancies after IUI have a higher incidence of low birth weight, prematurity, and perinatal mortality and morbidity compared to natural conception pregnancies	2a
Multiple pregnancies are the most important factor affecting the perinatal outcome after IUI	2a
The addition of ovarian hyperstimulation requires a strict follow-up of the IUI cycle to prevent multiple pregnancies	2a

TABLE 29.1

Statements of Chapter 29

Statement	Level of Evidence (LOE)
Patient Screening and Practices	
Infections originate mostly through biological specimens from patients that harbor infectious conditions, but can also occur through contact with health workers, contaminated laboratory environment, equipment, and storage vessels, as well as materials and supplies utilized during procedures	4
All biological specimens (blood and semen samples) must be handled with extreme care as a biohazard, since they are most likely to harbor infectious micro-organisms	4
A nonspermicidal condom should be used rather than the practice of coitus-interruptus, since the latter can result in the loss of the first sperm-rich portion and can contaminate the semen sample with vaginal flora and cells	3
Unnecessary prescription (costs and use) of antibiotics to male patients can be prevented, if comprehensive verbal and written instructions on laboratory procedures and guidelines on semen collection are provided prior to the initial semen evaluation, well before the scheduled IUI treatment cycle	3
Sperm Preparations	
DGC can be standardized and provide superior separation of highly motile spermatozoa from debris, leukocytes, and other cell types	4
Sperm samples contaminated with pathogenic organisms will negatively impact on IUI outcome	4
Sperm-washing techniques are used to prevent partner-to-partner transmission during an IUI procedure	2b
Sperm preparation techniques do not guarantee that HIV is 100% removed from the postprocessed sperm sample of HIV-positive males	2b
A ProInsert™ combined with DGC provide a biosecure method to purify spermatozoa from HIV-positive males	3
No seroconversions of female partners were reported in the literature, at this time, after inseminations with washed sperm from HIV-positive men	2b
Other	
Uncluttered work surfaces, hygienic working conditions, and waste disposal management will reduce the probability of laboratory contamination	4
Protective measures to adhere to while performing ART procedures are designed to protect laboratory personnel and certify aseptic conditions for gametes, zygotes, and embryos	4
Guidelines for good laboratory practices should be followed by trained personnel to promote quality and safety in the ART unit	4

TABLE 30.1

Statements of Chapter 30

Statement	Level of Evidence (LOE)
Sperm cryopreservation before cancer chemotherapy helps in the emotional battle against cancer	1a
Cryopreserved semen samples can still be used after more than 20 years of storage	1a
Semen cryopreservation is still not offered as a standard service in most centers treating male cancer patients	1b
Best IUI results with cryopreserved semen can be similar to IUI results with fresh semen	2a
Semen cryopreservation should be performed before the start of cancer treatment	1a
Cancer treatment has a permanent or temporary negative effect on semen parameters and males will seldom recover their full fertility potential after treatment	1a

TABLE 31.1

Statements of Chapter 31

Statement	Level of Evidence (LOE)
Sperm selection for IUI with gradients may result in increased probability for a certain gender, but the probability for the other gender is still significant	3
Sperm sorting using DNA binding compound Hoechst 33342 can increase the probability for the birth of a child with a specific gender after IUI but the probability for the other gender is still significant, especially when PGD is not possible to use	2b
The potential risks for DNA damage using DNA binding compound Hoechst 33342 have not been fully investigated	4

TABLE 32.1

Statements of Chapter 32

Statement	Level of Evidence (LOE)
There is widespread approval of preconception sex selection for medical reasons	4
Most international committees and many countries condemn sex selection for nonmedical reasons	4
Family balancing is frequently presented as a compromise between reproductive autonomy of the would-be parents and societal concerns	4

TABLE 33.1

Statements of Chapter 33

Statement	Level of Evidence (LOE)
The absolute pregnancy rate is higher with multi-follicular compared to mono-follicular growth	1a
CC + IUI is an efficient method of infertility treatment unless the insemination motile count is $<1 \times 10^6$ with a strict morphology score of <4%	2b
CC + IUI is associated with a low risk of multiple pregnancies and no moderate or severe OHSS	2b
There is no significant difference in clinical pregnancy rates between minimal stimulation protocols of CC + one HMG injection and conventional CC-HMG protocols used with IUI, while the first method is cheaper	2a
There is no significant difference in live birth rate between different methods of timing IUI	1a
There is no significant difference between conventional evaluation of sperm morphology and computer-assisted methods	2a
There is no significant difference in clinical pregnancy rates between different methods of sperm preparation	1a
There is no significant difference in live birth rates, clinical pregnancy rates, or the rate of miscarriages between soft and rigid insemination catheters	1a
There is no significant difference in clinical pregnancy rates between single and double inseminations in the same cycle	1a
In HIV infected semen samples, sperm washing and centrifugation on discontinuous gradients reduces the viral load to an undetectable level	2a

TABLE 34.1

Statements of Chapter 34

Statement	Level of Evidence (LOE)
IUI could be offered as a first-line treatment in case of nontubal factor, unexplained, and moderate male factor subfertility, provided the multiple gestation incidence can be reduced to an acceptable level and provided at least one fallopian tube is patent	1b
Multiple gestations are the most important complication associated with IUI after gonadotrophin stimulation and should be avoided as much as possible	2a
Semen decontamination through sperm processing can prevent transmission of life threatening STIs and other infectious agents, which constitute a high risk in developing countries and lower resource settings	2a

36

Summary: Grade of Strength of All Recommendations

Grade of Strength of Evidence Used in Recommendations (Guidelines)

A   Directly based on Level 1 evidence

B   Directly based on Level 2 evidence or extrapolated recommendation from Level 1 evidence

C   Directly based on Level 3 evidence or extrapolated recommendation from either Level 1 or 2 evidence

D   Directly based on Level 4 evidence or extrapolated recommendation from either Level 1, 2, or 3 evidence

GPP   Good practice point (GPP)

TABLE 2.2

Recommendations of Chapter 2

Recommendation	Grade Strength
IUI should be considered if the postwash TMSC lies between 0.8–5.0 million motile sperm	A
Screening for antisperm antibodies before the start of IUI could be of use	B
If tubal tests are performed, HSG followed by a diagnostic laparoscopy in case HSG shows no tubal patency is more cost-effective than diagnostic laparoscopy	B

TABLE 3.2

Recommendations of Chapter 3

Recommendation	Grade Strength
The prognosis of the couple should be taken into account in clinical decision making	A
The prognosis of the couple should be taken into account in the design of a randomized clinical trial	A

TABLE 4.2

Recommendations of Chapter 4

Recommendation	Grade Strength
In couples with a relatively good prognosis for spontaneous conception, IUI should not be started too soon	A
In couples with mild male subfertility with an average TMSC of 10 million, ovarian hyperstimulation should be added	A
IUI should not be applied when less than 0.8–5.0 million motile sperm are present after semen preparation	A
IUI can be applied in natural cycles in case of cervical hostility and probably in case of a moderate male subfertility	A
In couples with unexplained subfertility or mild endometriosis receiving IUI, ovarian hyperstimulation should be added. IUI in natural cycles should not be applied in these couples	A

TABLE 5.2

Recommendations of Chapter 5

Recommendation	Grade Strength
It is advised to add 2% albumine to the buffering medium upon sperm retrieval in case of immunologic infertility	GPP
In case of immunologic infertility IUI should be offered before starting IVF/ICSI	B

TABLE 6.2

Recommendations of Chapter 6

Recommendation	Grade Strength
In couples with unexplained infertility, IUI treatment should be limited to couples with female age under 40 years	A
No routine ovarian reserve screening prior to starting IUI treatment should be advised	B
When using donor semen, IUI may be encouraged to continue up to 42 years	A

TABLE 7.2

Recommendations of Chapter 7

Recommendation	Grade Strength
Men with a female partner above 35 years should be informed that increasing paternal age (40 years and above) has a potential negative impact on IUI success rates	A

TABLE 8.2

Recommendations of Chapter 8

Recommendation	Grade Strength
In women undergoing gonadotrophin-IUI treatment, the same BMI guidelines used for IVF cannot be applied	C
Recommending weight loss may not improve fecundity, but will improve obstetrical outcomes	B
The optimal BMI for natural fecundity may be between 20–24	D

TABLE 9.2

Recommendations of Chapter 9

Recommendation	Grade Strength
IUI should be used as a first-line treatment in case of moderate male subfertility provided more than 1 million motile spermatozoa are available after washing and at least one tube is patent	B

TABLE 10.2

Recommendations of Chapter 10

Recommendation	Grade Strength
Quality control and quality management in semen preparation for IUI is mandatory	GPP
Clinical outcome after IUI: there is insufficient evidence to recommend any specific SPT	A
Laboratory outcomes: the DGC is shown to be superior to the swim-up and wash technique	B
Novel sperm selection methods (based on sperm surface charge or nonapoptotic sperm selection) show promising results. However, they have not yet established themselves in routine practice, and their purpose for IUI is unknown; more evidence is needed	D

TABLE 11.2

Recommendations of Chapter 11

Recommendation	Grade Strength
More research is needed to investigate the importance of the time interval in IUI results	C
Since reducing intervals is inexpensive and risk-free, we recommend that times associated with IUI procedure are reduced, especially the interval between sperm collection and processing, which should be less than 60 min, preferably less than 45 min (LOE III)	C

TABLE 12.2

Recommendations of Chapter 12

Recommendation	Grade Strength
Couples with mild male subfertility, unexplained fertility problems, or mild endometrioses should be offered six cycles of IUI	A
Three cycles of IUI is the absolute minimum that should be offered	B
Young couples (below 35 years of age) should be offered the possibility to continue IUI up to nine cycles	B

TABLE 13.2

Recommendations of Chapter 13

Recommendation	Grade Strength
In an IUI cycle, if there is poor perifollicular flow (< 3 cm/sec) when the follicle is mature, consideration should be given to canceling the cycle	C
If more than three follicles have strong perifollicular flow (> 10 cm/sec), IUI should be canceled because of high risk of multiple pregnancy	GPP
A thick echogenic endometrium or a thin irregular endometrium before LH surge or hCG administration is an indication for hysteroscopy	A

TABLE 14.2

Recommendations of Chapter 14

Recommendation	Grade Strength
Timing of IUI can be performed with LH surge detection or hCG injection	A
Timing of IUI should be performed between 12 to 36 hours after hCG injection	A
In couples with unexplained subfertility, one adequately timed IUI is sufficient	A
In couples with mild male subfertility, double IUI should be performed in research setting	A
The frequency of insemination should not depend on multi follicular growth	A

TABLE 15.2

Recommendations of Chapter 15

Recommendation	Grade Strength
Women applying for TDI are not subfertile, while adding OH in TDI results in higher multiple pregnancy rates, we therefore recommend to start IUI or ICI in unstimulated cycles	C

TABLE 16.2

Recommendations of Chapter 16

Recommendation	Grade Strength
At least 10 to 15 minutes of immobilization should be applied after every IUI	A

TABLE 17.2

Recommendations of Chapter 17

Recommendation	Grade Strength
Mild ovarian hyperstimulation in combination with IUI should be applied in couples with unexplained or mild male subfertility and in couples with minimal to mild endometriosis	A
When ovarian hyperstimulation is applied one should strive after the occurrence of two follicles (using mild stimulation starting with 50–75 IU FSH per day) and gonadotrophins are the drugs of first choice	A
Aromatase inhibitors, GNRH agonists, or GNRH antagonists should not be used in IUI programs	A
Luteal support in ovarian hyperstimulation/IUI programs should be applied in randomized trials only	B

TABLE 18.2

Recommendations of Chapter 18

Recommendation	Grade Strength
Luteal phase support should be added to IUI cycles mildly stimulated with gonadotrophins in couples with unexplained subfertility	A
Luteal phase support should not be added to clomiphene citrate stimulated IUI cycles of normo-ovulatory women	A

TABLE 19.2

Recommendations of Chapter 19

Recommendation	Grade Strength
FSP can be used as an alternative treatment option for standard IUI in case of unexplained infertility and no Foley catheter is used	A
In case of unexplained infertility, a maximum of three FSP cycles is recommended	B

TABLE 20.2

Recommendations of Chapter 20

Recommendation	Grade Strength
PAF might be added to the IUI sperm wash procedure in couples with unexplained subfertility receiving OH/IUI; in couples with male subfertility, more studies are warranted	A

TABLE 21.2

Recommendations of Chapter 21

Recommendation	Grade Strength
Oral antioxidants given to infertile men with high semen OS result in significant reduction in semen ROS and serum Inhibin B levels, significant increase in the sperm linear velocity, and in the total, and per cycle IUI pregnancy rates	A
Use of oral antioxidants in male infertility found that these agents significantly improved the assisted (using *in vitro* fertilization and intracytoplasmic sperm injection) and unassisted conception rates and live birth rates and decreased sperm DNA damage	A
Repair of varicocele (condition which produces semen OS) is associated with higher pregnancy and live birth rates per IUI cycle than those who did not receive treatment	C
Use of antibiotic and anti-inflammatory agents for treatment of leukocytospermia is associated with significant improvement in pregnancy rates after IUI	B
Adding antioxidants to cryopreservative medium (e.g., vitamin E) during freezing significantly enhanced post-thaw total motile sperm and the percentage of progressive motility	B
No significant differences in pregnancy rates between the two sperm processing techniques such as density gradient centrifugation (DGC) and swim-up methods in the setting of IUI. DGC technique results in higher recovery rates of total motile, progressive motile, and viable sperm than the swim-up technique	A

TABLE 22.2

Recommendations of Chapter 22

Recommendation	Grade Strength
For couples with unexplained infertility first-line treatment with IUI with clomiphene citrate is cost-effective	A
The use of OH using gonadotrophins and IUI as an intermediate step prior to IVF has to be questioned, although recent data suggests equal efficacy to natural cycle IVF and IVF with elective single embryo transfer	A

TABLE 23.2

Recommendations of Chapter 23

Recommendation	Grade Strength
With sperm donation, couples and practitioners are pursuing the achievement of a healthy newborn with the maximum likelihood to succeed while also minimizing risk of transmission of infectious and genetic diseases or other undesired medical conditions	D
The main qualities to seek when evaluating potential donors are: first an assurance of good psycho-physical health status with confirmed absence of transmissible infectious and genetic conditions, and second, having an optimal sperm quality	D
Taking as reference the standards established by the European Union Tissues Directive, each country may include strict requirements regarding the infectious diseases to be screened in potential donors, as the U.S. Food and Drug Administration also states	D
A complete genetic history from the donor and his family is mandatory, and the donor should not declare that he does not have any major inheritable condition	D

TABLE 24.2

Recommendations of Chapter 24

Recommendation	Grade Strength
Single and lesbian women should be accepted in DI programs when professional counseling is available	D
The use of identity registered donors is strongly advised	D

TABLE 25.2

Recommendations of Chapter 25

Recommendation	Grade Strength
Adherence to guidelines for conventional fertility treatment and ART could alleviate uncertainty in patients	GPP
Clear information about reasons behind recommendation for conventional treatment will support patients' preference for this treatment option	D

TABLE 26.2

Recommendations of Chapter 26

Recommendation	Grade Strength
To prevent HOMP, prediction models can be used to select those patients with a good prognosis for a spontaneous pregnancy. Expectant management needs to be considered for this group	A
With mild stimulation protocols and monitoring most HOMPS can be prevented	A
When primary prevention fails, canceling IUI cycles or aspirating supernumary follicles are a low impact option for secondary prevention	A

TABLE 27.2

Recommendations of Chapter 27

Recommendation	Grade Strength
When combined with IUI, low dose gonadotrophins should be used instead of high dose gonadotrophins[a]	A
IUI combined with gonadotrophin treatment adjusted by nomogram is superior to standard dosing of 75 IU[b]	B
OH with IUI should aim for no more than two follicles[c]	A
Follicle aspiration can prevent multiple pregnancies while maintaining acceptable pregnancy rates[d,e]	B or C
In case of multi-follicular development, escape ART (conversion from IUI into ART) can prevent multiple pregnancies while maintaining acceptable pregnancy rates, when combined with single embryo transfer[d]	B or C

[a] From Cantineau and Cohlen, 2011, *Cochrane Database Syst Rev* 6:CD005356.
[b] From la Cour Freiesleben et al., 2009, *Hum Reprod* 24:2523–30.
[c] From Van Rumste et al., 2008, *Hum Reprod Update* 6:563–70.
[d] From McClamrock et al., 2012, *Fertil Steril* 4:802–9.
[e] ESHRE, 2009, *Hum Reprod Update* 3:265–77.

TABLE 28.2

Recommendations of Chapter 28

Recommendation	Grade Strength
When twins are to be prevented because of a higher perinatal morbidity and mortality, mono-follicular growth should be the aim	A
Preventive measures should be adapted if three or more follicles with a mean diameter of 14 mm or more are observed before ovulation/insemination	A
Couples should also be informed about an increased risk for perinatal health problems if they become pregnant after IUI	B
A pregnancy following artificial insemination has to be treated as a risk pregnancy	B

TABLE 29.2

Recommendations of Chapter 29

Recommendation	Grade Strength
Patient Screening	
Patients should be routinely screened for HIV, HBV/HCV as well as prevalent STIs in an IUI program, and laboratory staff should be notified of the test results, before processing or cryopreservation of any semen samples	D
Both male and female patients should be screened for pathogens and treated prior to an IUI attempt	C
ART units should consider the use of rapid tests in comparison to molecular assays for a first-line viral and STI validation	C
Sperm Preparations	
The sterile collection of semen for microbiological analyses and therapeutic use should always be followed	D/GPP
The risk-reduction sperm preparation procedures should be offered to patients that tested positive for blood-borne viruses (HIV/HCV/CMV) as part of an ART treatment procedure	B
A portion of the postprocessed purified sperm sample from HIV-positive males should be tested by RT-PCR for HIV-1 proviral DNA and RNA analyses, and only HIV-free samples should be used for IUI	C
High-security straws and dedicated liquid nitrogen storage tanks should be used to cryopreserve sperm samples after washing/decontamination	D
Healthcare Personnel	
Personnel should be vaccinated against HBV or viral diseases where vaccine is available	D
Ensure all staff are qualified and appropriately trained to handle infectious specimens	D
Protective measures should be enforced when handling body fluids (masks, gowns, and goggles)	D
Skin breaks on exposed skin of staff should be sealed with waterproof dressings and nontoxic powder-free gloves should be worn all the time	D/GPP
Environment/Procedures	
Laboratory facilities should be appropriately designed with adequate equipment and disposables to minimize various risks	D
Semen samples from patients who tested positive for blood-borne viruses should be processed in dedicated laboratory areas with appropriate safety measures	D
All procedures and manipulation of the semen samples for IUI should be performed in Class II biological safety cabinets with vertical laminar flow, using aseptic techniques and sterile disposables	D
All sharp objects should be handled with extreme care and rather be avoided when handling (semen and blood) samples from patients with blood-borne pathogens	D
Access to the laboratory should always be restricted, to protect the workplace integrity and to prohibit eating, drinking, as well as smoking within the laboratory	D/GPP

TABLE 30.2

Recommendations of Chapter 30

Recommendation	Grade Strength
Semen cryopreservation should be offered to all male cancer patients	A
Semen cryopreservation should be performed before the start of cancer treatment	A
Before semen cryopreservation, the patient should be counseled by a multi-task team	B
More research on semen cryopreservation is needed, especially for young adolescents and boys	B

TABLE 31.2

Recommendations of Chapter 31

Recommendation	Grade Strength
Sperm selection using gradients is not a suitable choice before IUI to avoid inheritance of serious genetic diseases	C
Sperm selection by flow cytometry sorting before IUI is not recommended as a means to avoid inheritance of a serious genetic disorder	B
Sperm selection by flow cytometry sorting before IUI is at present not recommended as a means for social gender choice (*family balancing*) since the risk for the individual without congenital factors is unknown but potentially severe	GPP

TABLE 32.2

Recommendations of Chapter 32

Recommendation	Grade Strength
The appropriate steps for introducing new techniques into the field of medically assisted reproduction should be started for preconception sex selection	D
Follow-up studies should be set up to determine the social and psychological consequences for the child and its parents of (a) allowing sex selection and (b) prohibiting sex selection	D
Studies should be organized to determine the social consequences for society at large, including the impact on ethical convictions such as the equality of the sexes	D
Public campaigns and educational programs should be established in gender-biased societies to address the social norms and structural issues underlying sex discrimination	D

TABLE 33.2

Recommendations of Chapter 33

Recommendation	Grade Strength
CC + IUI is an effective and affordable method for the treatment of infertility and is particularly suited to developing countries	B
Folliculometry + hCG should be used for IUI timing	B
Conventional semen analysis by trained personnel are as good as CASA for semen sample evaluation	B
In low resource settings, the simplest and most affordable sperm preparation technique should be used as it is as good as other methods	A
The simplest affordable catheter can be used for IUI as it is associated with similar pregnancy rates to more expensive catheters	A
A single properly timed insemination per cycle is sufficient and is as good as double insemination	A
In HIV discordant couples, semen samples should be treated with centrifugation on discontinuous gradients without fear of seroconversion	B

TABLE 34.2

Recommendations of Chapter 34

Recommendation	Grade Strength
IUI could be provided as a first-line therapy to all patients providing at least one patent tube and an inseminating motile count (IMC) after sperm preparation of more than 1.0 million	B
When ovarian stimulation is used, a careful monitoring of the IUI cycle is needed to avoid multiple pregnancies	C
Gradient techniques should be used in all settings with a high prevalence of STI/HIVs and/or a high rate of seminal infections	B

Index

T